EVEN GREATER
SEXUAL DISASTERS

Related books by Gyles Brandreth

Great Theatrical Disasters
The Bedside Book of Great Sexual Disasters

EVEN GREATER
—SEXUAL—
DISASTERS

GYLES BRANDRETH

Illustrated by Ed McLachlan

GRAFTON BOOKS
A Division of the Collins Publishing Group

LONDON GLASGOW
TORONTO SYDNEY AUCKLAND

Grafton Books
A Division of the Collins Publishing Group
8 Grafton Street, London W1X 3LA

Published by Grafton Books 1987

British Library Cataloguing in Publication Data

Brandreth, Gyles
   Even greater sexual disasters.
   1. Sex—Anecdotes, facetiae, satire, etc.
   I. Title
   306.7'0207   HQ23

ISBN 0-246-13199-3

Printed in Great Britain by
Robert Hartnoll (1985) Ltd, Bodmin

Contents

Introduction

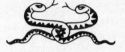

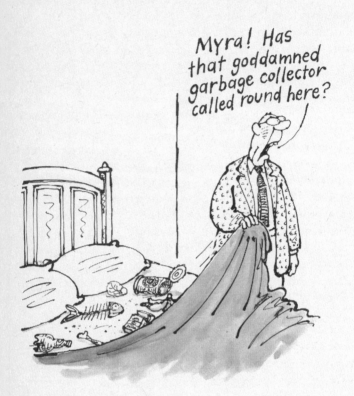

This book is packed with the most sought-after commodity of our times: safe sex.

Yes, join me between the sheets – these sheets – and you can have the time of your life, without a care or a condom. Here, at long last, is risk-free fun. In the pages that follow you can wallow in close encounters of the most lurid kind, let your libido loose on torrid tales of high jinks and low living, indulge yourself in clinches, clutches, couplings galore, and do it all in the certain knowledge that you'll emerge from this steamy, sensuous, sexy cavalcade of love and lust with your health and your reputation utterly unimpaired.

Even Greater Sexual Disasters is a catalogue of amazing, amusing and heart-warmingly appalling moments from other people's love lives. It is a consoling chronicle of connubial calamity and erotic catastrophe. What's more, it's a work you can rely on because it's written by One Who Knows. Let's face it, your author is a man who has lived. Even more to the point is that he's a man who has lived and loved and is ready to name names. Dear reader, I kissed Edwina Currie when she was a teenager.

You will find this volume rich in raunchy revelation. I've been squeezed by Diana Dors, I've held hands with Samantha Fox, for half a minute in 1965 I was in sole possession of Marlene Dietrich's left thigh. (I was helping her off the roof of her car at the time.) But I've not just larked about on the dolly slopes of the Everest of passion. I've been to the summit. It's not for nought that I'm known as Randy Brandy. Why only *yesterday* I made my way into the record books by sustaining the longest screen kiss in history!

Yesterday, since you ask, was Friday 13 February 1987, when on TV-am at just after half past eight in the morning Miss Cheryl Baker, the bedazzling star of Bucks Fizz, and I came face to face for three minutes thirty-three seconds, a remarkable osculatory encounter witnessed by millions and described by the London *Evening Standard* as having 'all the erotic charge of an over-60s church outing'.

Until yesterday the record for non-stop screen kissing was held by Jane Wyman and Regis Toomey who came lip-to-lip for 185 seconds in the 1940 film *You're in the Army Now*. My first attempt to outdistance the Wyman–Toomey mouth-to-mouth marathon was three years ago, again on TV-am, when I planted a solid and sustained smacker on the unsuspecting lips of the divine Anne Diamond. I have to report that Anne and I were trembling on the very brink of history when our smooch was cruelly brought to an abrupt stop by live coverage from Moscow of President Brezhnev's funeral.

Of course, given that yesterday's Baker–Brandreth can-oodle was a record-breaking triumph it shouldn't feature in these pages, and wouldn't were it not for the fact that Cheryl had a stinking cold and I've got it now. The price of yesterday's slurping is today's snuffling and I'll prob-ably have to go to the doctor and the dentist next week. Researchers at Adelaide University have shown that the lightest kiss can raise the heart-rate from 72 to 95 beats a minute and intimate kissing unfailingly spreads tooth decay.

If you thought kissing might be good for your health, think again. A student at Leeds University recently kissed her boyfriend and ruptured his eardrum. Another young lady, Miss Elizabeth Barry from Newhaven, Sussex, made the mistake of kissing the same fellow twice. On both occasions the kisses left her with lock-jaw. First time round, she spent two hours in the casualty department of the local infirmary as staff struggled to unlock her jaw. On the second occasion it took her six months to recover.

If a kiss and a cuddle can land you in hospital, is it any wonder that sex of any sort is rapidly becoming taboo? In the United States there is now an organization called Sexaholics Anonymous, formed for the salvation of those 'hooked on humping'. The founder is a psychologist, Patrick Carnes, who says, 'Sexual overactivity is no different from alcoholism. It's a disease.' He's against excess. He goes along with the poet who said it all in one of the briefest but most perfect poems in the whole canon of the literature of love:

> A little coitus
> Never hoitus.

'Moderation' is Dr Carnes's watchword. If you don't overdo it, you'll come to no harm. Clearly the worthy doctor hasn't heard about the clergyman from Broadstairs in Kent who led a life of exemplary moderation. Married to the same lady for a quarter of a century, ever-faithful to his wife, the vicar explained to the coroner that he and his good lady 'indulged no more than once a week, and never during Lent', but nonetheless on the occasion of their silver wedding their 'moderate love-making' caused their Jacobean four-poster bed to collapse, so killing the vicar's wife at a stroke.

The tragically widowed cleric was fifty-six, a dangerous age for lovers, according to Professor Jean-Paul Broustet of Bordeaux University: 'For a man in his fifties making love to his wife is as demanding as climbing three flights of stairs. But with a girlfriend, it is like sprinting five miles or racing up the stairs of a skyscraper.'

There are, of course, middle-aged men who could ascend the Empire State Building with a single bound. Sir Ralph Halpern, boss of the Burton Group and Britain's highest paid executive, is clearly one. I have before me the front page of the *People* dated 25 January 1987, where beneath the headline 'MODEL'S FROLICS WITH TOP TYCOON' a lovely young lady called Fiona tells all: '*Penthouse* pin-up Fiona Wright says that though she was just eighteen and he was a balding forty-eight-year-old, she could hardly keep pace with Sir Ralph's passion. She claims that during the twelve months she spent as his secret mistress the randy tycoon liked to play naughty games, spanked her in the shower, demanded sex up to five times a night, and kept his strength up by eating sunflower seeds.'

Whether or not the Wright revelations were wrong, they proved not to be the disaster for Sir Ralph that his friends and family at first feared. Indeed the Great Man's proclaimed prowess in the nookie stakes merely served to burnish his golden reputation as a potent entrepreneur. Shareholders weren't shocked: they were cheered to find that their leader was so evidently a man of action, energy and enterprise.

I have another recent newspaper in front of me which details the less fortunate exploits of another incredibly energetic individual. The paper is the *Star*, the date 11 February 1987, the headline 'THE STUD': 'A gigolo told a jury yesterday how he made a fortune from sleeping with wealthy women . . . and earned the wrath of his mother-in-law. Salem Mohammed, 33, said he had 3000 "clients", many middle-aged, some of whom paid him up to £10,000 for sex. The lusty lover said his wife Sehra did not object to his activities. But when her mother Doris Banks found out she was horrified.'

Well, it takes all sorts . . . You will find the highly-sexed in every walk of life, from kings to dustmen – literally. It is a verifiable fact that from the age of eleven until his death sixty-one years later King ibn Saud, father in every way of the Saudi royal family, slept with three different women a night – except during battle. At the other end of the social scale Harry Brown, a garbage collector from Ohio, didn't perhaps live so long (he died aged 59) but he claimed an average of four conquests a day over a quarter of a century – a feat of fornication that rivals the most remarkable scientifically-attested case on record, that recorded by sex researcher Alfred Kinsey of the man who averaged 33.1 acts of intercourse per week for thirty years.

Naturally, in a compendium of sexual disasters there's little room for the high achievers. This isn't the place for

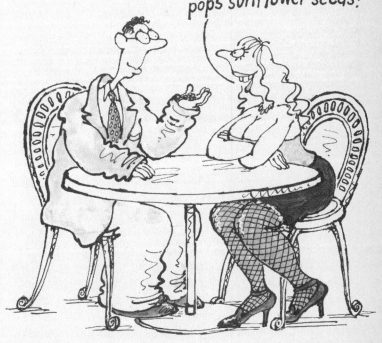

the ins and outs of how Mae 'I used to be Snow White, but I drifted' West once sustained fifteen hours of high-calibre intercourse with a fellow named Ted, however stimulating the saga. We're more concerned with the likes of Eddie 'I Gotta Big One' Johnstone, professional chemist and amateur Casanova who cruelly came a cropper when he entered the unofficial Sexual Olympics held at the University of California at Los Angeles in the summer of 1986. Ten-inch Eddie, as he liked to be known, was entered for the marathon event, where a prize of one thousand dollars was to be won by the couple who could sustain what the organizers choicely described as 'the longest quality screw'. Because of his awesome reputation, Eddie was excused the preliminary heats and given a bye to the final. From the outset he and his partner (Mrs Johnstone, as it happens) were clear favourites and entered the arena (one of the UCLA canteens converted for the occasion) with cheers in their ears and the scent of victory in their nostrils. Unfortunately when the starting pistol was fired, and the Johnstones prepared to strip for action, the unthinkable happened: Eddie caught his magnificent equipment in his zipper. Fearing that precious moments were being lost as her husband wrangled with his Wranglers, Mrs Johnstone intervened and with a violent jerk attempted to free her man's manhood. The effect was dramatic and painful, and resulted in 'I Gotta Big One' Eddie being rushed to hospital and the prize being carried off by a young couple from New Zealand who sustained their quality screw for just fifty-eight minutes but doubtless could have kept it up for hours had the proceedings not been abruptly halted by the unexpected arrival of the local police.

Indeed, throughout the compilation of this volume, the police have been most helpful with my enquiries. As often as not if it hadn't been for police intervention the case would never have come to court, and if it hadn't come to court it wouldn't have reached the pages of the press – and for collectors of sexual disasters newspapers are a prime source. Every day the press provides all the evidence any of us needs to support the claim that sex is dangerous. Look what I read in last week's *Sunday Express*: 'When sixty-five-year-old Henri Furnot discovered his wife Anna's affair with her hairdresser he shaved her bald and put her in hospital with a grazed skull.' And harken to the news from Colombo, as reported in yesterday's *Guardian*: 'Colombo has been suffering from a water shortage, but that did not prevent the fire department from pouring 5000 gallons of cold water on dozens of lovers in a city park. Wet and weeping girls and their boyfriends ran from Viharamahadevie Park on Wednesday after firemen trained hoses on trees and bushes. "A Wet Blanket on Park Lovers", the independent *Sun* newspaper said yesterday in a front-page story accompanied by photos of fleeing lovers. The fire chief, K. M. I. De Silva, was quoted as saying the move was meant to water shrubs and serve as "a deterrent to couples who are engaged in nefarious activities".'

And if the police don't get you, your partners will. Students of the popular press will have noticed that we've long passed the age of discretion. Anyone who's had anyone (and particularly anyone who's had everyone) is apparently now champing at the bit to Tell All – and in detail. Laid out before me is the sizzling centre spread from last Sunday's *News of the World*. Beneath the compelling headline 'I DITCHED MARIA (38D) FOR FLAT-CHESTED BILLIE (34A)' a torrid tale is told: 'Hunky male model Paul Kevin has given the elbow to the girl with the biggest assets in the Page Three business – for one who admits she is "flat as a pancake"! He has ditched Maria Whittaker, who weighs in with a stunning 38D bust, for skinny high-class fashion model Billie Muir. But what leggy Billie lacks outfront – her bust is near-invisible next to Maria's – she makes up for in brains. Paul admits: "Billie has no boobs whatsoever, but I love her." Maria has millions of fellows drooling over her charms, and they must think Paul is a lunatic for two-timing her. But he says: "Maria may have a fabulous figure but in bed she's not so hot. But Billie is a wildcat between the sheets." Modest Billie countered: "Well, it DOES take two to tango!" '

In the proper traditions of ruthless investigative journalism the *News of the World* gives the last word to Ms Whittaker's spokesperson: 'Maria's too much of a lady to get involved with a gold-digging wimp like him. She dumped him – because he was such a pain in the neck.' That's Maria's viewpoint and I can understand how she feels, though I'm here to tell you the lusty lad the *News of the World*'s important exclusive dubs a 'Romeo rat' is really rather a sweetie. I'd never heard of him till Sunday, but believe it or not, on Monday I met him. He and his dad came to put up some shelves in our dining room. That's the truth. I know nowt about his love-making, but his woodwork's impeccable.

The moral of all this is that having an affair with your hairdresser can make you go bald, making love in the bushes can lead to pneumonia, and over-familiarity with male models and carpenter's lads can land you bang in the middle of the *News of the World*.

I trust I've made my point. Sex is fraught with danger, but now you've *Even Greater Sexual Disasters* firmly in your grip you've nothing to fear and much to look forward to. As my father was wont to say, the recipe for a perfect night out is eating with a beautiful lady, drinking with a beautiful lady and going to bed with . . . a good book. I hope you enjoy this one.

Gyles Brandreth
14 February 1987

*Everything you
always wanted to know
about sex . . .*

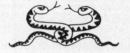

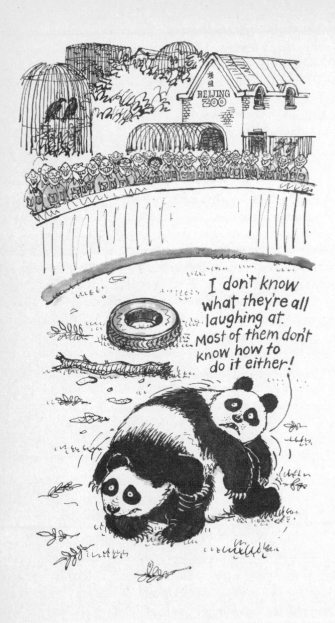

Victoria Wood once admitted, 'For a long time I thought *coq au vin* was love in a lorry,' and she probably isn't the only one to have made the same mistake. For something that is supposed to come so naturally, sex seems to cause more than its fair share of disasters. And far from helping, sex education sometimes has a lot to answer for . . .

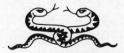

Witness the disaster that occurred when a church organist and Sunday-school teacher from Huddersfield decided to make his own sex education film for the benefit of the youngsters in his charge. In the home movie he was to portray Adam, and he persuaded a twenty-two-year-old member of the choir to give her all as his Eve. The film was shot in the early hours of a July Sunday morning in Huddersfield's answer to the Garden of Eden, the adventure playground adjacent to the municipal park. Unfortunately the epic was never completed, for Adam and Eve were arrested by a local constable after about half an hour of filming. They were charged with indecent exposure and stills were produced as evidence. The court agreed with the prosecution's contention that oral sex was not a feature of the Adam and Eve story as set out in the Book of Genesis and the couple were fined and bound over to keep the peace.

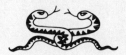

A rather more innocent epic on the same theme was contemplated recently by the Reverend Cyril Carter, vicar of Hounslow. With a forthcoming youth service in mind, he sensed that a film about Adam and Eve might find favour with the audience. It would have to be a film for real, he explained, 'you can't put Adam and Eve in trousers.' And he didn't.

Both leads were taken by nineteen-year-old students who appeared in the film naked as the day they were born. The only concessions made to artistic licence were the snake (Eve had a phobia about them and so the part of the serpent was taken by a sixteen-year-old schoolgirl – also starkers) and the location. It's not easy to recreate paradise in Hounslow. A private wood and some discreet corners of Windsor Safari Park had to suffice.

The Reverend Carter was careful to make sure that none of the parents of his potential audience objected to this unusual form of evangelism. 'We have been very careful with what shots we show and what is out of focus,' said the vicar, speaking with professional reassurance: he had taken it on himself to direct the film. He also took it on himself to destroy it before its screening, claiming that much of the publicity had taken the film out of context.

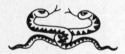

China has a steadily growing population of more than 1,000,000,000 – an indication that Chinese lovers know what they're doing, you might think. Not so, as a 1987 report revealed. Because sexual experimentation before marriage is a criminal offence, and because couples are forbidden to marry before both are in their mid-twenties, ignorance of the facts of life is rife. Sex education books are available, but to deter licentious readers they are sold only in packs which contain other 'useful' books, like guides to household carpentry or plumbing.

One young Chinese couple tried for two years for a baby without success before they began to suspect that they were doing something wrong. The problem? They had been lying beside each other night after night waiting for 'the molecule to jump from one person's body to the other'!

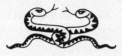

British children seem to have no such inhibitions, according to a recent survey in the magazine *Child Education*. Under the direction of Maurice Galton, Professor of Education at Leicester University, infant-school teachers were asked to comment on how their little charges were coping with the pressures of modern life – in particular, the extent to which they were copying adult behaviour. The results raised a few eyebrows.

One in three teachers reported that the Wendy house kitchen was becoming increasingly deserted as the mixed infants headed for the bedroom where they were discovered pretending to have sex with each other. The teachers showed surprising ingenuity in separating the little couples. One used to step smartly inside and announce to the writhing pair, 'I can hear the kettle boiling.' Another preferred to knock on the door and announce, 'It's Postman Pat – I've got a letter for you.'

But while parents and teachers are doing their best to steer their pre-pubescent children away from thoughts of sex, others are trying to encourage youthful awareness. In the course of a survey of artificial aids intended to boost a bust that nature might have skimped on, an article in the *Observer* suggested 'for the fairly flat who want to play it straight' a modest little number that went by the trade name 'Littlest Darling'. This is designed to fill an important gap in the market identified as 'ten-year-olds who are embarrassed at having nothing to show when they're changing for hockey'.

Schoolgirls aren't alone in their sexual anxieties. A survey conducted by the Nuffield Foundation into the sex habits of teenagers revealed that of the boys interviewed who possessed condoms, seventy-three per cent had never actually had sexual intercourse. Most admitted to carrying them as status symbols.

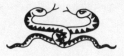

For many parents and teachers the decision whether or not to give sex education lessons is a difficult one. After all, if you tell children the facts of life they may well go ahead and experiment for themselves. The irony of the situation is not lost on the kids, as this quote, from a pupil at an early secondary modern school, indicates. 'The parson came to school and told us not to do it; the doctor came to school and told us how not to do it; and then the headmaster came and told us where not to do it.'

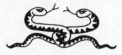

Once young people have the facts at their disposal many of them simply can't wait to get down to some serious practice. A father in Nantes, France, was checking through his fifteen-year-old daughter's schoolbooks when he came across a note from her biology teacher arranging a meeting after school. Suspicious, he quizzed the girl about her liaison and discovered what he feared – that she and her handsome young tutor were having an affair.

When he was summoned to the local police station the twenty-four-year-old teacher broke down and cried with relief at having been discovered. He explained how, after a series of sex lessons he'd given, he was approached by one of his female pupils who suggested that he might like to give her a more personal introduction to the subject. At first he'd resisted, but the temptation of a nubile and willing partner had been too much. Before long four of her friends demanded that he 'educate' them too, and when he'd refused they blackmailed him with threats to reveal all to the school authorities.

He was, he told the police and parents, absolutely shattered. What had seemed at first like a fantasy come true had turned into a nightmare. For nearly two months he had had a rendezvous with at least one of the girls almost every weekday afternoon. At weekends they had visited him at his home, sometimes three of them together, and demanded satisfaction. 'He was quite good in bed to begin with,' admitted one of his seductresses, 'but it got boring after a while. Now I prefer younger men.'

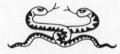

Not a sex education programme, though some children might be forgiven for the confusion if they'd heard this BBC schools broadcast . . . 'Now, are your balls high up or low down?' it started, and went on with, 'Close your eyes a minute and dance around and look for them. Are they high up? Or are they low down? If you have found your balls toss them over your shoulder and play with them . . .'

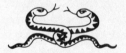

The US Medical Association has issued a word of caution to airline stewardesses seeking to put a little extra bounce into their work. Tests revealed that those who resorted to cosmetic surgery to improve their cleavage might find themselves up, up and away at cruising height. Apparently the silicone implants used to enlarge breasts have been known to explode at high altitudes.

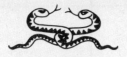

There are, of course, some problems which no amount of sex education can prepare people for. This letter was sent to *Oz* magazine in the 1970s by a reader who, for reasons which will soon become clear, signed herself 'Slap Happy'.

'Whenever my boyfriend and I have intercourse, during each stroke his balls slap against my body. In addition to this being painful for him, the slapping sound is so amusing that we have to momentarily stop because we start laughing. We have thought of taping his balls to his torso. Is there another solution to the problem?' *Is* there another solution?

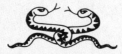

And in one of the more frank women's magazines there was a long correspondence about *this* reader's noisy problem. 'I seem to get air trapped inside me, so that when my current boyfriend and I make love I sound like a suction pump as it's expelled and then drawn in again. My last lover thought it was funny and liked to make the loudest and rudest noises possible, but the latest one doesn't seem to have such a good sense of humour and says he's never come across anything like it before. Is there anyone out there with the same problem?'

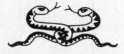

Never make love under a lorry – that was the sex lesson learned by students Hilary Cawdell and Steve Ashby when

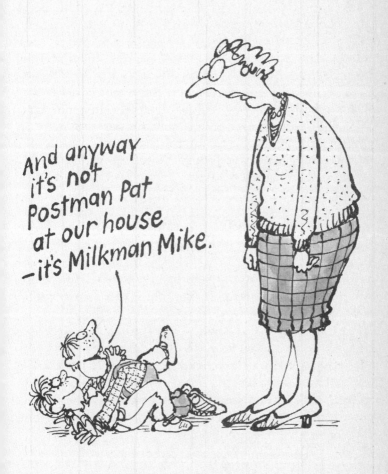

they were hitch-hiking across Europe. Arriving at the Swiss–Italian border late at night and in heavy drizzle, they decided to set up camp under one of the huge juggernauts parked by the side of the road. Having spread out their sleeping bags they were soon carried away; so carried away that they failed to notice when the lorry silently moved off, leaving them exposed in front of an appreciative group of truckers who gave them a round of applause as the performance reached its climax. Coming back from the local bar to spend the night in their cabs, the drivers had heard the couple's moans and had quietly let off the lorry's handbrake and pushed it a few yards across the car park so as to get a better look.

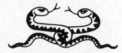

Napoleon Bonaparte's second wife, Marie Louise of Austria, must have had a fascinating surprise on her wedding night. Not only had she never seen a naked man before, she had never been permitted to look upon a naked male animal either! Equally surprised was a young Greek woman who jumped off a second-floor balcony on her wedding night rather than submit to the advances of her new husband. He jumped after her. She landed on a bush and was unhurt. He was killed. Protesting that she had been brought up never to let a man touch her above the ankles or below the neck, the weeping widow was taken back to her mother for a little more sex education.

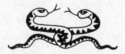

When it comes to discussing sex it's important that we all express ourselves clearly to avoid confusion. One worried reader wrote to *Mother* magazine: 'Usually the information given in your magazine is concise and accurate, but your article on circumcision left certain points uncovered . . . '

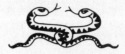

Consummating a Catholic marriage can be a tricky business if you don't know the right way of going about it, judging from an illuminating item that appeared some years ago in the *Irish Sunday Post*. 'No marriage is valid in canon law until it is consummated,' the article reminded its readers before warning, 'If any of *erectio*, *introductio*, *penetratio* or *ejaculatio* is absent – or if they happen in the wrong order – the marriage is not properly consummated and thus not valid.'

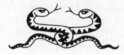

'I'm all in favour of sex education,' declared a lady writing to a women's magazine. 'Before I met my husband I didn't even know what a homosexual was.' Others, however, aren't of the same liberal turn of mind. One reader complained to the *Manchester Evening News* about the way corrupting information was being supplied to the public.

'In one of the "quality" morning dailies a doctor discussed the avoidance of cerebral thrombosis in middle-aged men. After a great deal of excellent advice he made the astonishing assertion that "making love", in terms of desirable energy expenditure, is the equivalent of a five-mile brisk walk. Quite apart from the fresh-air aspect, I do not think this sort of information should be available to the public at large.'

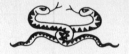

Others don't object to information, they simply don't want to have to give sex lessons themselves. A shy art teacher from Manchester admitted to her headmaster that rather than take a group of eleven-year-old pupils to the National Gallery for a school trip, as planned, they went to the Natural History Museum instead. In a note explaining her sudden change of plan she wrote, 'I took a party to the National Gallery last year and they spent the whole day making rude comments about the nudes and asking questions about anatomy and sex that I'm not prepared to answer. If you want them to go to the National Gallery you can send them with someone from the biology department.'

The Victorians knew all about the inflammatory effect of art on the impressionable young. In answer to an enquirer's question, 'How should I avoid the temptation towards sexual excess?', one nineteenth-century authority on these matters advised, 'Avoid the undue use of foods which are calculated to stimulate the reproductive nature. Use eggs and oysters, pepper and condiments with reasonable moderation. Do not stimulate impure thinking by theatre-going, the reading of salacious books, participation in the round dance, the presence of nude statuary and suggestive pictures.'

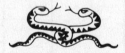

'I kissed my first woman and smoked my first cigarette on the same day; I never had time for tobacco since,' admitted Arturo Toscanini, proving that the woman who first introduces a man to the pleasures of sex gains a special place in his heart. Police chief Sergio Modini discovered how strong the attachment could be when he took over at a police station near Salerno in Italy. Determined to impose his authority, he ordered a total clean-up of the area. His officers dutifully booked all the minor traffic offenders they could find and hauled in petty criminals they normally turned a blind eye to. But when Modini himself led a round-up of local prostitutes, there was a riot at the police station. It was not the younger women the constables seemed concerned about, but one well-preserved lady in her fifties called Mama. They consoled her in the cells with espresso and cake while a deputation of officers was sent to see the new police chief and plead for clemency on her behalf.

Why, Modini wanted to know, should he bend the rules for one prostitute who was, quite frankly, old enough to know better? At this point one of Mama's supporters hit him and a brawl broke out. Only when it was over did someone have time to explain to the bewildered police chief that for three generations Mama had taken it upon herself to educate almost every boy in town in the arts of love. Most of the officers had been taken by their fathers to visit Mama for their first sexual encounter and all were so appreciative of her tender care that they threatened to resign *en masse* if Modini prosecuted her as a common prostitute. Tactfully, and perhaps remembering his own first time, the police chief dismissed all charges against her.

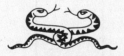

'I've only slept with the men I've been married to. How many women can say that?' asked Elizabeth Taylor. Pearl Thomson of Jacksonville, Georgia, certainly couldn't. She didn't sleep with either of her husbands!

Her first died tragically during their wedding reception after suffering a heart attack. Three weeks later, on the rebound, she married again and with her latest husband set off for the honeymoon hotel where she looked forward to her crash course in sex education. It was not to be. On arrival Pearl nipped into the bathroom to prepare herself for her first night of love – and found herself locked in. By the time the staff had managed to free her an hour later, husband number two had gone leaving only an apologetic note explaining that he'd got cold feet.

As the newly single Miss Olsen was interviewed by the press on the steps of the courthouse after obtaining her divorce she announced that she would be putting an advert in a contact magazine for a lover. 'I'm off marriage,' she told the news reporters, 'but I have no intention of dying the only twice-married virgin in the USA. I want a man who can teach me what my husbands couldn't.' The story doesn't end there, though, because one of the men who replied to her advert was – you guessed it – her second husband. According to the last report the two were living together in unmarried bliss.

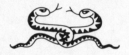

Three female Danish teachers were sacked after an angry mother discovered that the Physical Education course her son was attending at summer school would have been more accurately described as a practical sex education course. One of the teachers commented that she didn't understand what all the fuss was about – all the boys preferred the new sort of recreation to football.

Miss Vera Rainbird, a biology teacher from Sunderland, would have supported her Danish counterparts. After discovering her sitting on a desk with two naked sixteen-year-old boys at her side the headmaster of the school at which she worked fired her. Miss Rainbird took him to an industrial tribunal and claimed wrongful dismissal. The boys, she said, were simply helping her to give a demonstration about human biology, which she was teaching to the rest of the class. Her unorthodox teaching methods did not impress the tribunal and she lost her case.

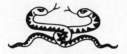

According to a 1987 report from one of the teaching unions, it's not women teachers who need to worry about classroom sex. Their research showed that forty-five per cent of male teachers had been harassed by girl pupils. Schoolgirls are not always subtle when it comes to the art of seduction. One south London teacher ran from his classroom when a pupil who had her eye on him began to peel off her blouse during a detention period. And on a geography field trip to Wales one good-looking young teacher had to be constantly chaperoned by another member of staff after a half-naked fifteen-year-old had crawled into his tent in the early hours of the morning.

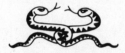

The Church Militant predicts that before too long there will be no need to teach sex education. In an article written thirty years ago it stated, 'In future when man learns to control his disordered impulses the time will come when the sex organs will atrophy and disappear and man will produce his kind from his larynx, which will be transformed to speak the Creative Word . . . Meanwhile we must make the best of a bad job.'

In her research on marathon runners, Susan MacConnie of Michigan University seems to have found evidence that supports *The Church Militant*'s prophesy. Ms MacConnie's investigations indicated that far from improving their virility, marathon nuts were in danger of losing theirs. She detected hormonal abnormalities which she reckoned might lead to shrinking balls. Next time anyone suggests you take up running you have your excuse!

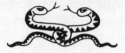

A little knowledge is a dangerous thing, as one pair of under-age lovers from Swindon discovered. Having decided that the best method of contraception would be the Pill, off they went to the family planning clinic. Everything seemed to be fine until the girl found that she was pregnant. They couldn't understand what had happened, she told the doctor.

Had she been taking the pills regularly? he wanted to know.

Not exactly, she admitted. Because she'd been frightened that her mother would find the packets, they'd decided that the boyfriend would take the Pill instead of her . . .

Some mothers are less careful about their daughters. One woman appeared in court in Romford in north-east London and admitted that she knew that her teenage daughter was having sex with a number of boys. 'It was just a phase she was going through,' she said dismissively.

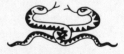

Bad news for those who like sun, sand, sea and sex on their holidays. Spanish cardiologists who were trying to discover the cause of the record 300 tourist deaths (one third of them British) in Majorca in 1986 have pointed the finger of blame firmly in the direction of afternoon nookie. Sex at siesta time, in the hottest part of the day and after a four-course lunch with plenty of wine, has been responsible for carrying off corpulent Casanovas by the dozen. 'The rest of the year,' explained Dr Jose Cortez, 'most north Europeans have a light midday snack and go back to work. But on holiday they let themselves go at the table and then tumble into bed with a partner. It is just too much for their hearts.'

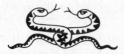

Some couples need sex therapy to make their marriages work, but for others it's a disaster. New York sex therapist Dr Richard Gunney was sued for divorce by his wife, who claimed that their marriage had been sexless for three years. 'If you worked at McDonalds all week would *you* want to eat hamburgers at the weekend?' protested Dr Gunney. 'I spend every day talking about sex and listening to other people's problems. The last thing I want to do when I get home is discuss more sex.' Mrs Gunney got her divorce. Dr Gunney moved to San Francisco and set up home with another sex counsellor who, we presume, understood his problem.

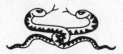

Despite the claims of some parents that sex education in schools corrupts the minds of innocents, those on the front line know that most children learn about sex, for good or bad, at home. A media studies teacher in Peterborough was discussing with her class of eleven-year-olds the ways in which advertising presented images of men and women. Tactfully guiding them away from the excesses of sexual exploitation and nudity, she set them a homework task of looking through magazines and newspapers and bringing to school pictures and stories about women. A week later more than half the class turned up with page three of the *Sun* and one child brought in two much-thumbed copies of *Playboy*.

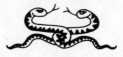

Finally, some people find themselves faced by dilemmas that no amount of sex education can help them solve. Take this letter from an understandably confused girl to *Woman's Own*.

'I've been going steady with my boyfriend for two years and we both intend getting engaged – we're both nineteen. He says he'll never marry a girl who's not a virgin and to be sure that I am one he wants to have intercourse with me before we become engaged . . .'

Baby talk

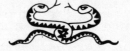

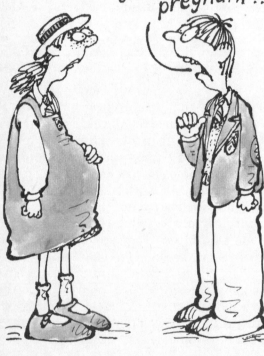

'It serves me right for putting all my eggs in one bastard,' said the inimitable Dorothy Parker on finding that she was pregnant. Accidental or planned, pregnancy and its results can lead to disaster . . .

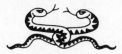

'I'm seventeen and expecting my fiancé's baby,' wrote one young lady to *Woman's Own*. 'We're planning to marry this year but he said if I were pregnant before our wedding day he'd never forgive me. I wouldn't like to hurt him by telling him I'm pregnant. What shall I do?'

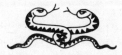

The five members of an all-male Wanganui sailing team were much more liberal-minded. During a competition in Auckland, New Zealand, they were introduced to lovely local model Linda Hadley. By the time they waved goodbye and set off home she had enjoyed the attentions of all of them, including three at once during a naked beach romp. When she discovered she was pregnant the five randy sailors agreed to take a blood test, but the results were not conclusive. Undeterred, they all decided to chip in to pay maintenance for baby Cheryl. 'We're good mates,' said a spokesman, 'and we always enjoy ourselves when we're away. This time we figured that it was fair if we split the cost five ways. We did think of holding a draw for the baby and whoever won could be her father, but for some reason Linda didn't like the idea . . .'

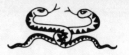

Many women faced with a baby but no husband must have been tempted to lay claim to a virgin birth. Investigations invariably prove a more mundane means of conception. However, an 1875 edition of the *Lancet* details a most unusual case.

'On 12th May 1863, a bullet fired in the American Civil War by the Confederates is said to have hit and carried away the left testis of one of Grant's soldiers. The same bullet went on to penetrate the left side of a young woman who was ministering to the wounds of the injured. Two hundred and seventy-eight days later, she, firmly insisting on her virginity, gave birth to an eight pound boy. The hymen was intact. Three weeks later Dr L. G. Capers of Vicksburg, Missouri, was called to see the boy because of a swelling of its scrotum. He operated and removed a smashed and battered bullet. He concluded that this was the same bullet that had hit the testis of the father, thus carrying sperm to the mother and fertilising her ovum.'

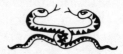

For those determined to avoid the patter of tiny feet, Glasgow Infirmary has the very latest in technology – a contraceptive bra. The bra is to be worn for nine days at the usual time of ovulation and detects vital changes in body temperature which it signals by turning green if it's safe to make love or red if it's dangerous. Presumably if it turns amber users should be prepared to pull out at any moment.

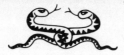

The contraceptive bra would have been welcomed by this couple who wrote to *Family* magazine in 1977. 'My wife and I knew nothing of the facts of life when we were married. And we were too shy to turn to our friends or anyone else for advice. We often wondered why our friends didn't have as many babies as we did, but we never dared to ask them. Looking back I must say that although we love our kids very much we wish we had asked.'

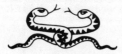

Maybe someone should have told them about Coca-Cola! Investigations by Harvard Medical School reveal that throughout the Third World, Coca-Cola is used as a contraceptive douche. Experiments indicated that it is surprisingly effective. Ordinary Coke killed 91 per cent of sperm and Diet Coke was even more effective, killing 100 per cent. However the new formula, widely introduced in 1984, was only 42 per cent successful. The Coca-Cola company has no plans to exploit the contraceptive powers of its product, however. 'We make no claims in this direction,' said a spokesman.

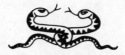

If a fizzy douche doesn't appeal, how about the diaphragm? According to the *International Herald Tribune* a few years ago 'A long-term study of contraceptive methods is highly favourable to the diaphragm, with researchers finding no material risks other than pregnancy . . .'

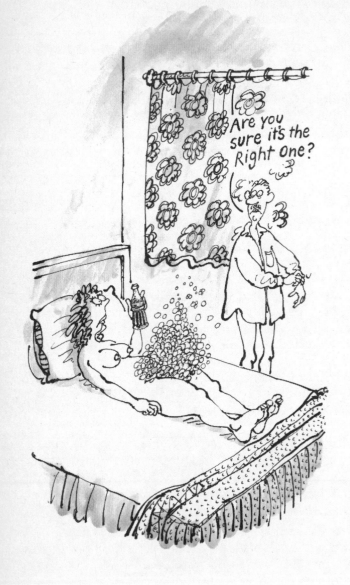

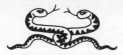

Throughout history people have used an amazing variety of substances for contraceptive purposes. Elephant and crocodile dung, lemons and clay are just a few. In her autobiography *An Unfinished Woman*, the author Lillian Hellman recounts a story of her Aunt Jenny, who was asked by a young woman how she could avoid pregnancy. Aunt Jenny advised drinking a glass of iced water before sex and taking three more sips during the act. Some years later Lillian Hellman wrote to her aunt to tell her that she was about to get married. By return came a telegram reading:

FORGET ABOUT THE GLASS OF ICED WATER TIMES HAVE CHANGED.

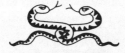

Johann Ketteler didn't fancy a stint of national service in the West German army, so when he was called up for a medical examination he took with him a sample of his girlfriend's urine. He knew he'd be turned down because she was a diabetic. It took a week for the sample to be analysed and then Johann received another call to the army medical centre. He went along cheerfully and was delighted to hear from the senior pathologist that tests on his urine had indeed revealed an abnormality. His satisfaction was short-lived. The doctor told him he was pregnant.

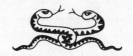

Health and fitness fan Horst Petry wasn't pregnant but he was determined to breastfeed his baby when his wife announced that she was going back to work six weeks after the birth. A course of hormone tablets allowed him to develop the necessary equipment and he successfully fed his son before weaning him on to an organic vegetarian diet. Unfortunately Mrs Petry didn't appreciate Horst's desire to bring up baby. Claiming that he was unreasonably obsessed with natural living and motherhood, she applied for a divorce. She got it, too, but her husband got the baby. In his summing-up the judge commented that he had never before met such a dedicated or concerned father but that he thought Horst should lay off the hormone tablets.

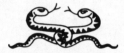

A Philadelphia news report told the tale of Mr Frank Speck, who had a vasectomy only to discover several months later that his wife was pregnant. She decided to have an abortion, which was duly performed. Not long after that she gave birth to a baby girl. Both Specks are suing both doctors.

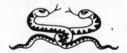

Some people go to extraordinary lengths to avoid having babies. Others do extraordinary things to get them – sometimes with devastating results. Vasili Liandros, a young Greek working in Wolfsburg, West Germany, was shattered to learn that he was sterile and that his wife Maria would never have his baby. Ever resourceful, Vasili approached his neighbour Klaus Weilmann, who was married and already had two children, and asked him if he would be a surrogate father. Klaus agreed, accepted a fee of £2000 and got down to completing the deal with Maria.

After six months of trying, and with no indication of a baby on the way, Vasili suggested that he should see the specialist who had diagnosed his own problem. The result was unexpected; Klaus was sterile too. From there things could only get worse. Not only did his wife admit that their two children had been fathered by another man, but Vasili started proceedings to sue him for breach of contract.

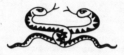

Television has been blamed for leading to permissiveness but rarely has its use as a contraceptive been acknowledged! Not so long ago the *Sunday Mirror* carried this letter from one wife. 'We find most programmes absolutely boring but we dare not switch off. On the two occasions the set broke down I became pregnant. So now we watch until the white spot disappears or one of us has dropped off to sleep.'

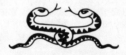

We all know that nurses aren't paid enough for the work they do, but no one was aware of how hard up they really were until a Wigan hospital administrator revealed that no fewer than thirteen nurses working in his hospital had become pregnant the previous year for the sole reason that they had felt obliged to pay their boyfriends back for dinners and nights out that they couldn't afford themselves.

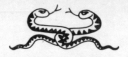

Disaster can strike even when you're totally innocent, as Toronto father-to-be Carl Martin discovered. Many women develop strange cravings when they are pregnant, and Carl's wife was no exception. She was addicted to a particular brand of minty toothpaste. Early one morning Carl woke up to find her pacing, distressed, around the bedroom. She'd just finished the last tube of toothpaste and she was desperate. A more considerate husband would be hard to find. Carl called the local drugstores but couldn't find any open, so as a last resort he threw on his bathrobe and went to ask the neighbours in the apartment upstairs if they had any toothpaste to spare.

His neighbour's attractive wife answered the door and couldn't have been more helpful. She brushed aside Carl's apologies for disturbing her sleep with the news that her husband was working overnight and invited him to come in while she searched the bathroom cabinet. After a few moments he heard her calling him and followed her into the bathroom – where he found her sitting naked on the side of the tub, a tube of toothpaste in her hand. He was welcome to it, she smiled enticingly, but she was going to require a rather special form of payment. Carl wavered for a few seconds, knowing how desperate his wife was. Alas, they were a few seconds too long, for at that moment the lady's husband returned. Unimpressed by the story of the toothpaste he knocked Carl cold before throwing him down the stairs. Mrs Martin was so upset that by the time the ambulance arrived to carry Carl off to hospital she had started labour, and while he was being treated for cuts, bruises and concussion she gave birth to their son.

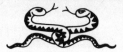

Lou Hunter from Santa Monica spent five days in a Los Angeles hospital while he was treated for an eye infection. Ten days after arriving home the hospital accounts department sent him a bill for three hundred dollars for the delivery of a baby. 'Please correct the error,' he wrote back, 'or at least send me the baby.'

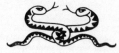

When Dorothy Parker received the news that a friend's wife had given birth she sent the following telegram:

DEAR MARY, WE ALL KNEW YOU HAD IT IN YOU.

And when Norma Shearer and Irving Thalberg had a son Eddie Cantor sent them this message:

CONGRATULATIONS ON YOUR LATEST PRODUCTION STOP SURE IT WILL LOOK BETTER AFTER ITS BEEN CUT.

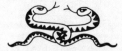

This little story is reported as having happened in places as diverse as New York and Milton Keynes, but that doesn't mean to say it isn't true! According to most versions, a hotel chambermaid lets herself into what was supposed to be an empty room and discovers the deputy manager, a man she knows to be married, making love most enthusiastically to a very pregnant stranger. Covered in embarrassment the couple lie there blushing while the chambermaid waits for an explanation. At last the deputy manager blurts out, 'It's all right, she's my sister.'

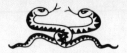

Sex and showbusiness have always been natural bedfellows but seldom so strikingly as in the case of a Women's Institute group in Mason City, Iowa, which was forced to cancel its production of the play *World Without Men* because every member of the cast – seven women and a cat – had become pregnant.

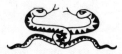

Newcastle Social Services Children's Committee were interviewing a woman in her twenties who had four children by the same father. During the course of the interview one of the children's officers enquired if there was any particular reason why she had not married the man. 'I didn't like him enough,' she was told.

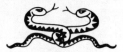

Australian apiarist Eric Mason was crazy about children – and that had unexpected consequences. Eric and his wife Lorna had seven children whom they raised on their bee farm beside the Murray River. To give them a hand with the domestic chores they employed a girl named Jean. Before long Jean had become a part of the happy family, and when Eric and Lorna moved to another farm after three years, Jean and her four children by Eric went along too. To maintain harmony and make everything official, Eric decided to marry Jean and the open-minded Lorna acted as the witness. With eleven junior Masons running riot around the place, Lorna and Jean decided that extra help was needed and Ruth, an English girl, joined the household. She also joined Eric's private harem. It wasn't long before Eric decided to do the decent thing and marry her too. This time Jean cropped her hair off, put on Eric's clothes and took his place for the wedding. Ruth's tally of children was three. There might easily have been more domestic help and more Masons had the neighbours not kicked up a rumpus at the growing tribe. Subsequent investigations revealed the unorthodox family structure and Eric was sent to jail for five years.

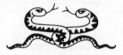

Men can be terribly sensitive about their fertility. Would-be fathers working in Haringey Council's offices in north London were alarmed to receive an official-looking letter advising them to wear copper-reinforced underwear as protection against dangerous low-level radiation being beamed at them by their computer screens. It could make them sterile, the letter warned. While some worried chaps went straight to the local shopping centre to try to purchase the necessary protection others contacted their union, which revealed that the whole thing was a joke.

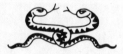

Marie Stopes, British birth control pioneer, took the problem of male fertility seriously too. Her belief that trousers rubbed and damaged the genitals must have made her own son's sex life a disaster. She insisted that he wore a kilt or a knitted skirt of her own design.

Getting to
know you . . .

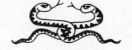

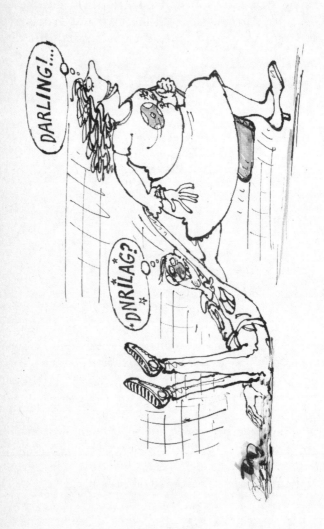

'Make love to every woman you meet; if you get 5 per cent on your outlay, it's a good investment,' advised Arnold Bennett, who must have had plenty of practice at seduction. Sex and seduction go hand in hand like love and . . . well, marriage. And like love and marriage the gentle art of seduction can lead to some dramatic disasters . . .

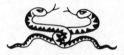

It pays to be sensitive about the sexual likes and dislikes of your partner. A Glasgow man was raced to hospital after his reluctant girlfriend sank her teeth into him as she performed fellatio. 'She was never very keen,' he was reported as saying. 'I suppose oral sex is a matter of taste.'

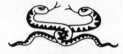

Sally Ann Cooper from St Cloud, Minnesota, treated herself to a shopping trip to Minneapolis and called in for a haircut at a chic salon run by two dark-eyed Latin hairdressers. During the course of her visit, she later explained to a jury in the state courthouse, she was forced to commit indecent acts with both men before the senior partner took her into a back room, removed what remained of her clothing and had his way with her. Meanwhile the other stylist totted up her bill and asked her for twenty-five dollars before she left. Did she pay this? asked the judge.

'Of course I paid it,' snapped Ms Cooper.

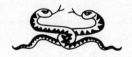

Some people go to extraordinary lengths to get to know the person they think is for them. Attractive model Blanche Blair appeared before a judge in Sacramento, California, charged with her twenty-fourth speeding offence in ten months. When he asked how she came to be in the dock yet again, Blanche blurted out, 'I've fallen in love with you and don't know how else I can see you. Can I have your photograph?'

'Request denied,' growled the judge, pounding his gavel, and the besotted Blanche was fined $50.

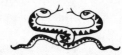

It didn't take long to get to know glamorous and amorous Romanian Vera Renczi. Lusty local men in search of a good time found that it was easy to arrange clandestine meetings with her. Unfortunately Vera had an unusual habit; she killed off her lovers one by one and kept them in zinc-lined coffins in her basement, along with those of two of her husbands and a son, as mementoes. One of her favourite pastimes was sitting among them after dinner each evening. By the time the authorities caught up with her there were thirty-five coffins in her collection.

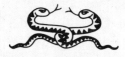

'Give a man a free hand and he'll run it all over you,' Mae West warned – and knowing Mae West she probably didn't mind if he did. But Nelly Kranks did mind when the plumber she'd called in to fix a burst pipe suggested that she pay him with a kiss. She hit him over the head with a spanner from his own tool kit and then turned the blow lamp on him. And just in case he hadn't got the message, she kicked him out of the house and down a long flight of stairs from where he crawled into the street begging for mercy.

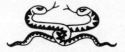

The music scene is famous for its sex and drugs and rock'n'roll, but as one groupie discovered, all is not necessarily what it seems . . . Her letter to *Melody Maker* reveals what *really* goes on among the wild boys of rock.

'I travelled round with a group and praised their music and watched their every action,' she wrote. 'I helped the lead guitarist stick stamps in his album. Then one horrible night, as I was walking down a dark alley, the boys set upon me. They held me on the ground, removed every single piece of my clothing and then, grinning lecherously, they stuck Ban the Bomb stickers and World Cup stamps all over me. It was horrid. I can never now live a happily married life, because every time I see my husband's priceless collection (he's got several penny reds and a jubilee issue) I just pass clean away. So please, rampant group members, control yourselves.'

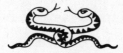

A young man from Taiwan who fell madly in love and wrote seven hundred letters to his sweetheart discovered the bitter penalty of too ardent a passion. She married the postman.

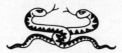

Teenage passion was the cause of one of the worst traffic jams ever experienced in Rio de Janeiro. While traffic lights changed and the cars around hooted, the loving couple remained locked together in a front-seat kiss. For two-and-a-half hours they embraced. Then police fought their way through the irate motorists and discovered the cause of the problem. A dentist was sent for and before long he'd managed to disentangle the young lovers' dental braces.

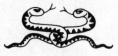

'Love me, love my dog,' goes the saying, and Birmingham bachelor Paul Simmons didn't think there would be any problems when he met art teacher Carol Kurtz and her three Alsatian dogs – after all, he liked dogs. But no matter how much he loved Carol, he couldn't make the dogs love him. On their first night together Paul was stunned to find that Carol shared her bedroom with her pets and that as far as *they* were concerned nothing had changed. After a romantic dinner together he and his new love retired to bed and the dogs came too. Undeterred by the three pairs of eyes watching every move the loving couple got down to business. Unfortunately the dogs misinterpreted Carol's sighs of pleasure and came to her rescue. Paul was badly bitten around the back, neck and buttocks and spent several days in hospital recovering and deciding whether love was worth it.

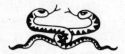

Other men have a less persuasive way with them as this letter from a disgruntled young lady reveals. 'Men have strange ways of showing affection. For instance, a boy I have known for five years has hardly ever used my real name, calls me Old Pip, Catsmeat, Dogsbody, Fishface, Horace, Mole and many others in the same vein. No wonder girls are left asking, "Is this love?"'

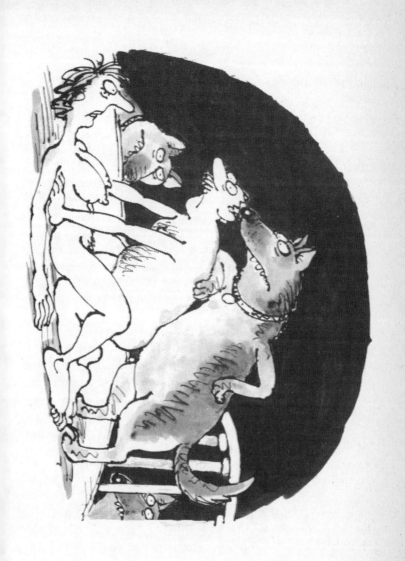

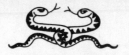

There are, of course, some men who are determined to do things properly, whatever the cost. Gary Austin from Vancouver researched women's magazines for helpful hints on how to seduce his girlfriend. When she arrived for dinner at his apartment she was delighted to find it full of flowers, lit by dozens of flickering candles and with perfume and soft music wafting through the air. A specially made heart-shaped dessert clinched the matter, and before long they tumbled into bed together.

They were still hard at it when firemen broke into the bedroom, dragged them apart and carried them draped in sheets down a ladder to safety. In their hurry to get to bed they hadn't bothered to extinguish all those candles.

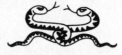

Englishmen have never been the romantic kind, and Englishwomen have grown resigned to the fact. Even so, this advert from an East Anglian newspaper must be the ultimate in anti-romantic proposals.

'Owner of tractor (on H.P.) wishes to correspond with Widow who owns a modern Foster Thresher, object matrimony; send photograph of machine.'

And what kind of woman would feel compelled to reply to *this* desperate plea in the *Beckenham and Penge News*? 'Man 45, 6'2", fed up with being one of the boys, wishes to meet woman 40–50 who feels the same.'

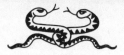

Sex-starved Welsh lovers Lisa Santacroce and Robert Jones searched every cranny for nookie. Unable to find a home together, they finally rented a garage and installed a double bed so that they could spend some time in private. But after two weeks of unbridled passion they were evicted by the local Bridgend council, following complaints by passers-by that they could hear everything that was going on inside. According to councillors, garages are for parking, not larking.

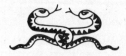

Clark Gable may have been a perfect lover in the dreams of millions of movie fans around the world, but there were several leading ladies who did all they could to avoid close contact with the King of Hollywood. Vivien Leigh was one of them. After winning the part of Scarlett O'Hara from a field of more than 1400 hopefuls, she couldn't have been too thrilled to discover that her Rhett Butler wore smelly false teeth which he seldom cleaned, and that his breath was like a distillery. And she didn't fare much better with another heart-throb, Marlon Brando, in *A Streetcar Named Desire*. In real life Brando was apparently as boorish as his screen character, Stanley Kowalski – definitely not the kind of man to appeal to Miss Leigh. He soon got the message and went out of his way to grunt, belch and fart whenever she came near. To avoid this, she spent most of the time in her dressing-room, pressing her gloves.

Joan Crawford had similar problems with dashing matinee idol John Barrymore, who not only had bad breath but also refused to shave. At the end of a long day's shooting his leading lady's face was covered in a red rash caused by his bristles. Errol Flynn's reputation as a womanizer cut no ice with Olivia de Havilland during the filming of *Captain Blood*. Despite all attempts to win her heart she refused his affections. Perhaps it's not surprising when you consider that one of his methods of seduction included leaving a dead snake in her panties.

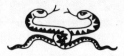

Even in Shakespeare's day actors were sex symbols. Richard Burbage was playing *Richard III* one night at the Globe and so captivated one female member of the audience that she went backstage during the interval and invited him to her home for a good time after the show. Shakespeare overheard the plans for their assignation and nipped out of the theatre before the final curtain to beat Burbage to bed. The lady must have been happy to accept the Bard as a substitute lover because they were hard at it when Burbage arrived, announcing himself as Richard III. When this information was brought to the lady's bedroom, Shakespeare told the maid to give the answer that William the Conqueror had come before Richard III.

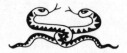

Desire can strike in the most unexpected of circumstances, as Lee Jaques discovered on a trip to Disneyland when he took an immediate shine to the unlikely figure of Minnie Mouse, who was at the gates greeting people. Lee, from Rugby, lunged at her while the seventeen-year-old employee inside the costume did her best to fend off his advances. Security guards came to her aid and Lee spent five days cooling his ardour behind bars at the Orange County Jail.

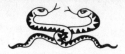

After divorcing his wife of more than forty years, Florida millionaire Arnie Taylor decided to look round for a new partner. His first wife having been naturally dark, he resolved to go in for a change and put an advert in a contact magazine for blonde ladies under thirty who might like to become Mrs Taylor number two. Fourteen women replied and Arnie, unable to decide, dated them all and then held second-round auditions in bed. That was where disillusionment set in. On more intimate acquaintance he discovered that only five of them were natural blondes. 'They were nice girls but I don't feel I could trust a blonde now,' he announced. 'I'm going to see if I can't find a nice natural redhead.'

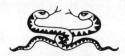

When it comes to seduction, persistence pays off – that was the theory of Antwerp office Romeo Fred Hartmann. Having set his heart on a new secretary in the marketing department, Fred visited her office every day, left her notes, waylaid her on the journey home from work, called her at weekends and spent every lunchtime hanging around trying to persuade her to come out with him. For three weeks she refused him, but at last his hard work paid off and she agreed that he could come to her flat one evening.

He couldn't believe his luck when he turned up with a bottle of champagne under each arm and found her waiting, smiling, for him. Before long they were exchanging kisses on the sofa in her sitting room. Then she got up and went into the bedroom, telling him to follow her when she called him. Expecting to find her waiting naked and eager for him, Fred removed his own clothes and, when the call came, sprang ready for action into the room.

Alas, it was not to be his big night. Waiting for him were all the other women from the office whom he'd tried to seduce. They handcuffed him, tied a bright pink bow tightly round a now deflated part of his anatomy, and dragged him out of the building on to the street, where they chained him securely to a lamppost at the side of a main road. By the time the police arrived to cut him free, Fred admitted that he'd got the message.

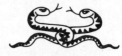

It's not always men who won't take no for an answer. Bristol solicitor Terence Allen was sitting at his desk in October 1986 when in burst a thirty-eight-year-old woman, demanding to marry him there and then. The wedding was booked for midday, she announced, and the wedding car was waiting outside. Then she handed him a note stating her proposal in writing.

This wasn't the first time that Jennifer Mogford had popped the question. Only the day before she'd been bound over for pestering Mr Allen, who was already married himself and had recently handled her divorce. Her past exploits had included chasing the object of her desire around his garden and badgering his secretary to recall him from his holiday in Brazil. Asked to account for her unusual behaviour in court, she explained that she had lost custody of her two children during her divorce and she thought that she would stand a better chance of getting them back if she was married.

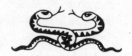

If demands by politicians and church leaders for a return to old-fashioned values alarm you, take heart from a story that was said to have taken place in the 'naughty' 1890s. At that time house parties, held in some of the smartest English country houses, provided ideal opportunities for guests to get to know one another – and not just over the breakfast table. During one particular party, held near Petworth, the glamorous host and hostess decided to play a practical joke on their guests. *She* made secret assignations with most of the men, telling them that they were to come to her at two in the morning; she would place a marker outside the door so that they would know the coast was clear. With each of them she arranged a different signal – a handkerchief, a flower, and so on. Meanwhile her husband was making similar arrangements to visit the ladies.

The evening passed with dinner and dancing and lots of excited and anticipatory glances and at one o'clock everyone found an urgent reason for retiring for the night. Then the host and hostess put their plan into action, placing the pre-arranged signals outside the ladies' doors. At five minutes to two, unable to wait any longer, the first gentleman tiptoed from his room, followed soon after by the others. The host and hostess waited in anticipation for the cries of confusion – but they were denied their joke. The bedroom doors stayed shut while the bewildered but nevertheless eager couples made the best of the mix-up!

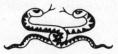

A man caught in another man's wife's bedroom has to think pretty quickly of an excuse. For anyone contemplating adultery, this could be a useful story. Lord Cardigan had slipped into a lady's bedroom during a house party, convinced that her husband was miles away, when in he walked. As he blustered, Cardigan silenced him with, 'Sh . . . Don't wake her. I was passing . . . thought I smelled smoke, but all's well!' and slipped away leaving the husband at an even greater loss for words.

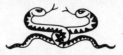

What are the three vital ingredients for a successful singles cruise? At a guess I'd say single men, single women and a ship. The cruise advertised by the Malchi shipping company and the Click matchmaking service also offered a trip round the Mediterranean, luxury cabins, swimming-pool, first-class food and an on-board psychologist to help the socializing, so it was no wonder that bookings for the *City of Rhodes* flooded in. The problem was that all the applicants were women, and the cruise had promised equal numbers of single men and women.

With the money in the bank and the ship in the harbour Malchi and Click thought it would be a pity to cancel the holiday and disappoint so many people, so off they all sailed. They could hardly have been out of sight of land before at least fifteen single ladies formed the rapid conclusion that they'd been fleeced. There wasn't a solitary single man to be found aboard; worse, they were marooned on the ship for another seven days with dozens of other single women. Anyone searching for the psychiatrist, as well they might under the circumstances, was in for a disappointment too. He hadn't made it aboard.

Once back on dry land the fifteen furious ladies headed straight for their lawyers and sued for £3500–£1000 for their wasted money and the balance in damages for their mental suffering. Not surprisingly, neither of the two companies concerned tried to defend themselves.

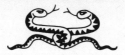

They say love is blind – and it's even more blind when the lovers have never seen each other, as a young Italian farmer from the Canneto district of northern Italy discovered when he resorted to a marriage broker to find a help-mate and wife. Before long he was writing to a girl from Canecatti in Sicily, who fulfilled all his criteria except for one – she never posted him a photograph, 'because there is no photographer in our village'. When the two met for the first time the would-be groom understood why. If everyone in the village looked like his pen-friend, there wouldn't have been much call for one.

The girl's family were quick to sense that he had lost interest and explained that since he'd promised to marry her in writing she was now 'compromised'. In fact they made it quite clear that it was an offer he wasn't going to be allowed to refuse. The only way of getting round the problem was to find another man willing to take her on. When last heard of the farmer was offering a million lira to anyone willing to marry her, and no one had responded . . .

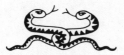

Perhaps he should have taken the kind of drastic measures employed by another jittery Italian. Ello Brazzale was so nervous about getting married that he robbed a house on his way to the church in the hope of being caught and missing his wedding. It worked, and he was arrested as he walked up the aisle in Vicenza . . .

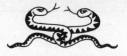

Sexual attraction is a matter of taste, as this young lady realized after a disastrous party.

'I went to a dance which was started off with the guests being given a label bearing the name of half a well-known dish. You had to find the person with the other half. For instance, fish went with chips, roast beef with Yorkshire pudding, and so on.' So far, so good. Then a hint of uncertainty creeps in as she discovers that her label reads 'egg' . . . 'I found a boy labelled bacon, but when I spoke to him he said, "Let's have a look first." Then he went off with a girl labelled liver and I was left with nobody except a boy labelled onions . . .'

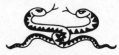

Felipe Jax was first introduced to his wife Linda after he mugged her in Las Vegas. Linda, a black belt karate expert, felled her attacker with a flying kick as he made off with her handbag. Then she sat on him while someone called the police. But for both of them it was love at first punch and by the time the cops arrived, mugger and victim had run off hand in hand. 'I really like physical men,' said Linda when the police eventually caught up with them.

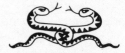

Karen Bowen thought she'd met the man of her dreams in a Windsor nightclub. They danced and drank together and then he drove her back to his large house on an expensive new estate. Upstairs in the master bedroom suite Karen forgot her inhibitions and romped in the jacuzzi before giving her all to the lucky fellow on the king-size bed. When she woke up the next morning her wealthy Romeo was nowhere to be seen – but three strange faces were peering at her from the end of the bed. One was the estate manager, the other two were customers who'd come to inspect the show house.

Games
lovers play

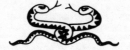

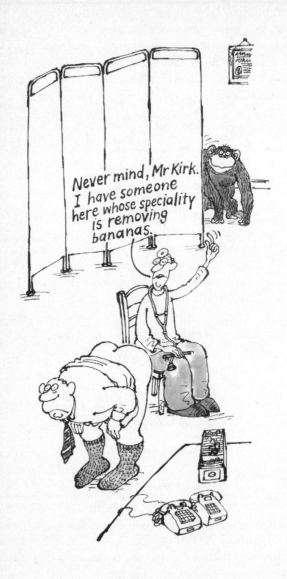

'I felt a bat's squeak of desire,' admitted the Earl of Gowrie after watching Edwina Currie MP brandishing a pair of handcuffs at a Tory party conference. Thank goodness the noble Earl felt nothing stronger, for the one sure way to beckon calamity into your sex life is to try an unusual diversion. Whether it's a new position or a sex aid, leaving the straight and narrow in the pursuit of the kinky can be fraught with peril . . .

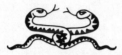

Middle Eastern terrorists were planting bombs all over Paris, so when postal sorter Georges Fermat, who worked in the main post office in Dijon, picked up a parcel addressed to a Mlle Natalie Dupont and found it was ticking he called in the bomb squad. While the post office was being evacuated, police swooped on Mlle Dupont's flat to see what she knew of the package. To her acute embarrassment she knew quite a lot. There wasn't a bomb inside the parcel, she explained, but a battery-operated vibrator which she'd sent away for and which must have been switched on in the post . . .

And while we're on the subject of vibrators and embarrassment, doctors at St Bartholomew's Hospital have recorded a new sexual trend. Within the space of a fortnight two male patients were rushed into the accident and emergency department suffering from, in medical jargon, 'a painful vibrating umbilicus'. Further investigations showed that both were homosexuals who had formed close attachments to their battery-operated dildos. In each case the devices had disappeared inside at the moment of climax, leaving the patients vibrating, humming and in great discomfort. The vibrators were retrieved without great difficulty; after all, doctors are used to removing far more weird and wonderful things. A list of retrievals published in one American medical paper included a large bottle of glue, an orange, a toy rocket, a pencil and a banana . . .

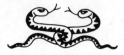

Even more embarrassed than people rushed into hospital to have a banana removed from a place where a banana should never be was the husband of a British Airways air hostess. She made regular short-haul flights from Heathrow airport, which suited her husband whose particular pleasure was to be tied up and locked in the bedroom wardrobe while she flew to Paris and back. Disaster struck in August 1984 when the plane on which she was due to return was grounded. Faced with an unscheduled overnight stop the frantic air hostess had no alternative but to call the police and request that they break into the house and rescue her husband.

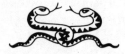

Help came too late for another German with an unusual habit. He was found seated on the loo, stark naked and with, of all things, a potato masher firmly entangled round his privates. Enquiries revealed that he had discovered that this particular kitchen utensil provided a sexual thrill all of its own. With a little adjustment he was able to connect it to the lamp socket in his loo and was in the habit of locking himself in regularly for his favourite shocking pleasure. Exactly how he came to discover this invention will never be known, for one fatal day he was sitting on the loo enjoying himself when he reached for the lavatory chain before switching off the masher at the mains. The chain formed a direct earth; there was a flash and a puff of smoke and he was electrocuted.

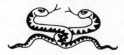

Potato mashers are not the only household appliances that have been put to unusual use. Steve Cox (yes, really) from Norwich had to be rescued by the fire brigade after getting his penis trapped in a bath tap. He wouldn't explain how it happened and I don't intend to speculate here. Another major domestic risk for men is the Hoover. The *British Medical Journal* has highlighted Hoover problems on several occasions.

There was the London man who was admitted to hospital for repairs to his genitals after, he told them, the Hoover had mysteriously turned itself on and sucked him in while he was changing its plug. Staff were sceptical; how many people do you know who change plugs in the nude? Across the Atlantic a Denver man found himself in the same predicament after hoovering his car wearing nothing but his underpants. According to him the Hoover had got blocked up and he was only trying to free the blockage, using a somewhat unorthodox part of his anatomy, when it suddenly started up. In seconds he found part of himself gumming up the works. Stitches and skin grafts were required to repair him.

The lesson is obvious. Stay away from Hoovers, especially when you're naked!

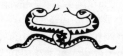

'Bisexuality immediately doubles your chances for a date on Saturday night,' according to Woody Allen, but it can also double your sexual hang-ups. Take this case, for example . . .

Having been dressed as a girl for the first five years of his life, a young medical student grew up with an enthusiasm for women's lingerie and clothing. At the age of twenty-three he asked to be castrated and later had plastic surgery to make him a woman. However, within a couple of months his male sexual instincts returned and he was lusting after female students. Only a few weeks later the plastic surgeon found himself undoing his original work and restoring as much as he could of the patient's equipment. Everything seems to have turned out fine and the student, definitely a 'he', is now a pathologist.

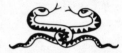

Sex changes are more common than many people imagine. A burglar who broke into a Streatham house in November 1978 found the occupant, an attractive blonde woman, at home. Instead of fleeing he chose to woo her, and within thirty minutes of sweet talk attempted his first kiss. Unfortunately the object of his desire responded with a right-hand punch, a left-jab and a half-nelson. How was he to know that prior to her sex change operation she'd been a bricklayer?

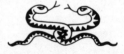

Anxious to inject some spark into a dull marriage, a Californian couple purchased themselves a video camera and went off for a week's holiday to a Santa Barbara hotel. Instead of taking pictures of the local scenery they spent their time filming themselves making love in a variety of positions and playing back the very blue movies using the TV set in their room. They enjoyed this form of home entertainment so much that they watched themselves night after night. When, exhausted but happy, they packed their bags and came down to the reception to pay their bill on the last day, they were stunned to discover a dozen of the hotel staff waiting for them with flowers and champagne. Even better, the manager waived half their bill. What, they asked, had they done to deserve such treatment? It was only then that they were told that their home movies had been relayed to every TV set in the entire hotel and that the staff and some of the guests had been glued to the newest channel all week!

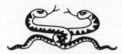

People with bizarre sexual preferences have problems in finding suitable partners or assistants. The members of a pagan sect based in south London are a case in point. 'Sex is one of our most powerful tools,' explained their spokes-man. 'For many of our rituals we require a virgin of seventeen summers. Unfortunately, it's getting more and more difficult to find them in Eltham these days.'

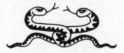

'Men who aren't pet lovers aren't any good in bed,' according to Jilly Cooper. According to American sexual research around five per cent of the male population have proved themselves to be pet lovers in the fullest possible sense. The most common objects of their desires were sheep, calves, donkeys and dogs in that order, though a surprising number had had their way with hens. They are not alone in their liking for feathered friends; the Chinese were renowned for the way in which they petted their geese. In Islamic desert societies a man's best friend is without much doubt his camel. Another piece of American research investigates the most unlikely creatures to be involved in bestiality and comes up with live snakes and fish, both of which have been used by women as replacements for men.

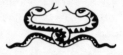

Less exotic, but equally strange, are the things which can turn an ordinary heterosexual on. A man from Arizona wrote to *Forum* magazine to share his problem with its readers; he could only make love to girls who limped. His letter was prompted by a recent experience when he'd fallen madly in love with a female tennis player who'd sprained her ankle. While she hobbled around wearing a bandage their sex life had been great, but as soon as she was better he simply couldn't rise to the occasion, not even if she faked a limp.

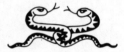

The Germans are known to like their women big and sporty, and Reinholdt Bauer, who was only 5 feet 2 inches tall, was no exception. He used to haunt the red light district of Hamburg looking for the biggest partner he could find. He eventually discovered his ideal woman in a flaxen-haired, 6-foot, 24-stone Brunnhilde of a lass who satisfied his every whim, including sitting on his face. It was this particular peccadillo that finished him off; he suffocated.

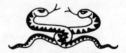

The physical punishments used in English public schools

have been held responsible for the peculiarly British obsession with whipping, beating and humiliation. Among those who developed a taste for the cane at school were Doctor Samuel Johnson, famous wit, moralist, philosopher and dictionary compiler, who never forgot the thrashings he'd received as a boy at Lichfield Grammar School. He kept a set of padlocks and fetters in which his friend Mrs Hester Thrale would confine him while she applied the rod.

Victorian poet Algernon Swinburne was even more addicted to the kiss of the whip. Numerous floggings at Eton determined his sexual preferences at an early age and he was a regular client at a brothel in St John's Wood which specialized in such discipline. He even wrote poems about it. One of them, 'The Flogging Block', came complete with annotations by one Barebum Birchingham. His friend and fellow poet Dante Gabriel Rossetti once gave actress Adah Menken £10 to seduce Swinburne. She did her best but had to give the money back to Rossetti, saying, 'I can't make him understand that *biting's* no use . . .'

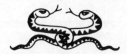

Not so long ago an understandably anonymous man was taken into a London hospital after a whipping session with his mistress. She, reluctant at first to ply the birch as hard as he'd requested, had soon developed a taste for the work and overdone things. Hospital staff reported that although he'd had to have stitches he was vowing that as soon as they'd healed he'd be back for more.

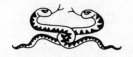

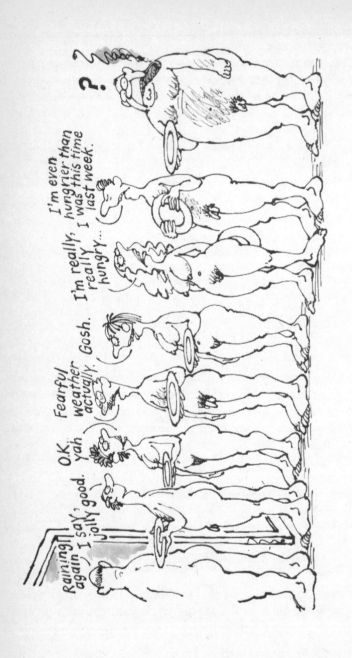

Anyone who chuckled at the antics of guests at Mrs Cynthia Payne's south London parties will know that while British orgies are not always sophisticated or glamorous, they're fun. Apparently this hasn't always been so. Al Goldstein, editor of *Screw* magazine, reported that British orgies are more formal than those held elsewhere in the world. 'Soon as I arrived I was told to take my clothes off and queue up for my food,' he reported of one party. 'The hostess insisted that we ate everything up before the orgy. I don't feel people were enjoying themselves much.'

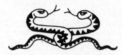

Some of the practical problems involved in group sex were highlighted in a magazine feature about a club in New York that used to specialize in orgies. Female guests complained that there was no secure place to leave their handbags while they enjoyed themselves, so they took to carrying them into action. This created its own problems, including that of bag snatching while the ladies' minds were on other things. Eventually secure facilities were arranged, but that didn't solve the problem of glasses. Short-sighted guests who needed their specs to size up potential partners found that in the heat of the moment their glasses were going missing – and more often than not they were rolled on and damaged in the general frenzy. After a spate of insurance claims for ruined lenses, guests were asked to leave their spectacles with their clothing.

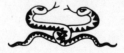

It's not on record whether the members of Catherine the Great's sex club wore glasses or carried handbags during their orgies at the Hermitage. Led by the sixty-year-old queen, whose appetite for sex had increased over the years to match her huge frame, more than a hundred people at a time would participate in the elegant surroundings of the royal palace. Unfortunately the exclusive nature of the club soon began to tell; so many women of the court contracted VD from male carriers that a secret hospital with room for fifty patients had to be established.

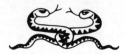

The fourth Marquis of Hertford liked to make sure he got value for money in everything – including sex. When he paid Napoleon III's mistress the Contessa di Castiglione a million francs for 'one night of love, without excluding any erotic refinements' he made sure she earned every penny of it. Such were his lordship's demands that she had to spend the following three days in bed before she could stagger uncertainly to her feet.

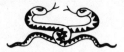

'There is no unhappier creature on earth than a fetishist who yearns for women's shoes and has to embrace the whole woman,' wrote Karl Kraus. Islington shoe-fancier Ronald George perfected a way of getting the shoes without having much to do with the women. His main tactic was to stop women in the street and offer to clean their dirty shoes for them. The moment they stepped out of their footwear he raced away with his prize. When he was really desperate he went as far as stopping women motorists and telling them they had an oil leak which he could fix with the heel of their shoe! By the time he appeared in court he'd stolen shoes worth more than £689.

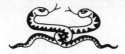

A fetish of a different sort put the phantom bra-thief of Workington in the dock. More than a dozen housewives in the Workington area complained to the police of having their underwear stolen from their washing-lines, but the case was solved only when a vigilant member of staff at a local department store caught the thief in the act. Seventy-two-year-old Alfred Morris pleaded guilty to trying to leave the store with four underwired and two natural-form bras in his pockets. When police searched his home they found another forty bras in a cardboard box in his greenhouse. Mr Morris claimed that he intended to fill the bra-cups with potting compost and propagate seedlings for his garden in them. He normally used pots he bought from the garden centre but was no longer able to afford them, he explained. The judge sympathized and said that he appreciated that these days it cost a small fortune to keep a garden looking good, but fined Mr Morris nevertheless.

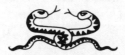

As fetishes go, shoes and bras are pretty tame. A nameless man from Deal in Kent probably thought that his desire to be cased from head to toe in black latex was fairly harmless, too. He sent away for a fetching all-in-one rubber suit complete with a zip at groin level and a face mask which he'd seen advertised in a Sunday newspaper. When it arrived he eagerly ripped off his own clothes, rubbed himself with talcum powder and squeezed himself slowly into the suit. Once clad, with the zip strategically open, he began to realize that all was not well. The wrists and the chest of the suit were so tight that they began to cut off his blood supply and restrict his breathing. With growing alarm, he found that no matter what he did he couldn't get the garment off.

In panic, and unable to do up the zipper, he lurched into the back garden where his next door neighbour's wife was working. She screamed at the sight of this extraordinary flasher, threw her secateurs at him and ran back to the house where she locked herself in and dialled for the police. They arrived just as the rubber fan was about to pass out and promptly cut him out of his precious suit. Far from evoking a grateful thank-you, this action enraged him and he threatened to sue them for the cost of his lethal outfit. That was the point at which they arrested him for indecent exposure . . .

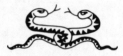

Also guilty of indecent exposure were two young German lovers who came unstuck – or, more accurately, *stuck* – while making love in Bremen docks. Whether it was the fault of the cold, damp atmosphere or just the girl's nervousness no one could tell, but after her lover had come he simply couldn't go. No matter what he did, his girlfriend had him gripped tight in a strong muscular spasm she couldn't control. They remained locked together and unable to move until a crowd of delighted onlookers gathered and eventually called an ambulance. Once at the hospital the girl had to have chloroform before she could be persuaded to let her lover go. He was extricated and suffered nothing worse than bruised pride and privates.

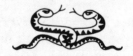

Suffering from bruised pride and a sore finger was jolly gigolo Heinrich Bronn who bought a parrot, hung its cage over his bed and taught it to say 'Wonderful, oh wonderful!' whenever it was asked the question 'How was that?' One night Heinrich lay back after making love to his latest lady and asked her, 'How was that?'

The parrot missed its cue and instead of answering properly gave a vulgar laugh. Angry that the joke had been spoiled, Heinrich reached up to give the dozy bird a prod. The parrot bit his finger off.

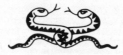

You don't have to resort to rubber, leather, whips or even parrots to bring immediate disaster to your love life. Ingrid Grazsteuer, yet another German, decided to give her husband a little shock and see whether it would spur him into sexual action. Hiding in their bedroom one night, all she did was greet Helmut Grazsteuer with a piercing shriek that wouldn't have been out of place in a Wagner opera. Poor Helmut panicked, made a wild dash for safety, tripped over a stool and crashed through a window. The bed in which he spent the next six days was in a hospital ward, not Ingrid's bedroom.

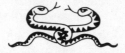

Perhaps Ingrid would have done better to use an aphrodisiac in her attempts to revive Helmut's interest – though not all aphrodisiacs live up to the claims on the packets. 'Span-Fly' was marketed as the modern version of an age-old aphrodisiac, Spanish Fly, and its makers claimed that one dose would be guaranteed to unleash explosive desires in even the coolest of lovers.

One man, finding himself in need of a boost, bought

six packets and swallowed the contents all at once. The only explosions he experienced were those of chronic flatulence. Nothing happened. He called in his local trading standards officer who had the 'Span-Fly' analysed. It was composed of citric acid, caffeine and bicarbonate of soda.

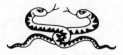

Another sexual charlatan was quack clergyman Dr Graham, who opened a Temple of Health and Hymen in Pall Mall. The biggest selling point of the place was its Celestial Bed for Superior Beings, which was claimed to restore lost sexual urges and vigour and to help childless couples. For £100 a night – a quite astronomical sum at that time – his clients could lie back on a mattress stuffed with stallion's hair and containing 1500 magnets while music played, incense wafted and naked girls danced round the bed. It didn't work, of course, but it must have been an amazing sight!

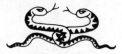

There must be *some* aphrodisiacs that work – if only you can get hold of them. In 1499 Cesare Borgia married the sister of the King of Navarre, Princess Charlotte d'Albret. To make his wedding night a memorable one for them both he ordered a supply of aphrodisiac pills. Unfortunately for him, some joker thought it would be amusing to substitute them with laxatives. He spent the night not, as planned, coming, but going – to the loo.

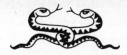

Jimmy 'The Beard' Ferrozzo didn't need to take pills or potions or other aphrodisiacs. He worked at the Condor Club in San Francisco, alongside one of the most erotic topless dancers on the West Coast. Just watching her act was enough to turn most of the male clientele on. At closing time one morning Jimmy and the dancer found themselves alone in the club and decided to put their relationship on a more intimate footing – on top of the club's grand piano.

Jimmy weighed sixteen stone (225 pounds) and his passionate exertions rocked the piano to such an extent that it triggered the mechanism that raised it all the way to the ceiling. When the cleaners arrived several hours later they found Jimmy crushed to death between the piano lid and the roof beam, still astride his lady love who had survived the encounter apparently unscathed – aided perhaps by the fact that she was so drunk she couldn't remember getting on to the piano in the first place.

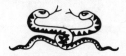

Death at the piano might have been an appropriate end for two Czech composers Janaček and Kotzwara, but in fact both died enjoying themselves in bed. Music reference books state that Janaček died in the arms of his mistress, but what most of them fail to explain is that they were in bed together and hard at it at the time. The seventy-four-year-old composer applied himself *allegro con brio* but found that his heart could only answer *diminuendo*. A requiem followed.

Kotzwara's end was even more colourful. He had a penchant for elaborate forms of bondage. On the night he died in 1793 he persuaded a London prostitute to truss him up so completely that he was left dangling from the ceiling and entirely helpless. In the past it had always been arranged that he should be cut down after hanging in this state of ecstasy for five minutes. Unfortunately on this occasion he was left too long, and his 'friend' was left with the task of explaining to the police how she came to be in possession of a dead body.

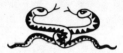

But of course, some people wouldn't recognize the trappings of a bizarre sex life if they tripped over them. A courier with a travel firm told a Sunday magazine about a group of pensioners she'd escorted on a tour of Scandinavia. They spent a day in Copenhagen, and after they were safely back at their hotel two elderly ladies took great delight in showing her the smart black leather harnesses they'd bought for their dogs back home. Did she tell them that the ritzy harnesses were in fact intended for bondage purposes? Of course not. And I bet the dogs didn't give a damn either.

Marriage
lines

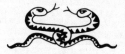

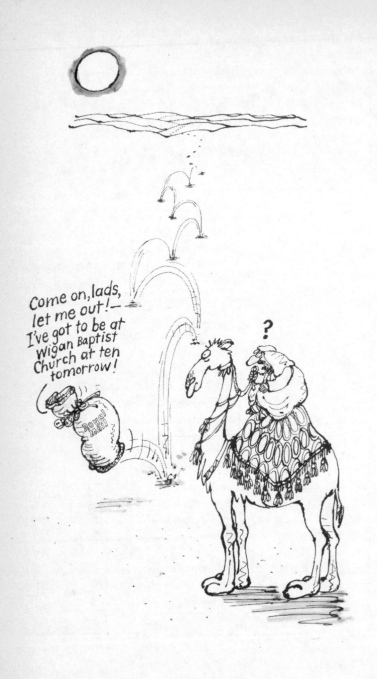

'All marriages are happy,' observed Raymond Hull. 'It's the living together afterwards that causes the trouble.' The problem with some marriages is that the participants have different ideas of what to expect from wedded life. Take Somerset Maugham on the subject. 'A man marries to have a home, but also because he doesn't want to be bothered with sex and all that sort of thing.' Is it any wonder that for many people disaster is already lying in wait as they walk up the aisle?

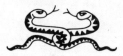

One way of avoiding the problem of marrying in haste and repenting at leisure is to take your time over things. Joe Fonge and Elizabeth Allen did. They had their first date in the small Oxfordshire village of Holton in 1917. By 1967 Holton had changed quite a lot and so had the shy lovers who at last, after half a century of courting, found the courage to tie the knot.

It took only forty years after the partition of India in 1947 for Wazifullah Khan, a shoemaker from Pakistan, to track down his fiancée Khursheeda. The couple had been about to marry when politics and history swept them aside, split their country in two and left them looking for each other for four decades.

Gertrude Horn and Philip Edwards had to wait almost as long, and all because of old Mrs Edwards who didn't see eye to eye with her future daughter-in-law. 'She was the only obstacle,' said Gertrude. 'It would have meant living with my mother-in-law, and she made it plain that she would have been the boss in the house. I wasn't having that.' So she decided to wait until Mrs Edwards went to meet her maker. At the age of seventy-six she married her man.

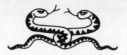

Alan and Glynn Lambert spent their first night together behind bars. As they drove from Harrogate to Lyme Regis and their honeymoon hotel, their car blew a gasket on the A40. They spent the next two hours shivering on the hard shoulder until a police patrol car arrived to rescue them. By now it was late and the officers confirmed that extensive repairs would be needed before they could complete the journey. However, anxious to preserve the romance of the occasion they put a radio call through to the nearest police station in Witney, and by the time the hapless honeymooners arrived a vacant cell had been transformed into a bridal suite complete with a four-foot-wide bed, mattress and four blankets. The newlyweds spent their first married night together while the cells around them echoed to the snores of a poacher, a supporter of Swindon Town football club who'd been arrested for being drunk and disorderly and a stray Pyrenean mountain dog.

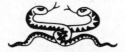

Stag nights have terrific potential for disasters. One bridegroom only just made it to church on time after being trussed up in a mailbag and put on board a train bound from Stafford to London by his friends. They thoughtfully supplied a return ticket which he was able to use after being rescued by startled railway workers.

An Irish bridegroom who couldn't swim missed the ceremony completely after being marooned in a rowing boat in the middle of a lake. His friends rowed him out there the night before, dropped anchor, then jumped out and swam to the bank, taking the oars with them. They arranged for one of their number to go and collect him a few hours later, but by that time all the rescuer could think of was his hangover. It was only when he failed to turn up at the church that they remembered where they'd left him.

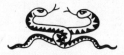

A line-up for the title of Most Disorganized Bridegroom would have to include Brian Delisle-Tarr who set off for his registry office wedding without a ring because he hadn't been able to get to the jewellers. Realizing that he was going to have to improvise if the lovely Angela was to be his bride, he lifted the bonnet of his car and removed a jubilee clip from one of the hoses. At the appropriate moment in the service he slipped this makeshift token of their everlasting love on to her finger and pronounced the immortal words, 'With this jubilee clip I thee wed.' Instead of solving the problem this only made the disaster worse. The jubilee clip became stuck fast on the bride's finger and she had to be driven to the local fire station to have it removed.

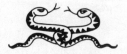

In America they have a different way of doing things. With the flinging of lawsuits almost a national pastime, there's a growing movement towards drawing up pre-marital contracts and laying out the ground rules before a couple walk down the aisle. One husband-to-be demanded a guarantee that his mother-in-law would not be allowed to live in. Another refused to get married until his model-slim fiancée had signed an agreement that she would forfeit rights to alimony if she put on weight and he left her. Wives have insisted that their careers be given equal consideration in family plans and one extracted a promise that her husband would do the washing-up, help with the housework and carry out the rubbish. There are some who have made their men swear to give up smoking, divide the cupboard space in any home down the middle and even turn vegetarian. Before Aristotle Onassis and Jacqueline Kennedy were married they negotiated a 170-point contract!

Not everyone agrees that this is the right way of ensuring happiness. Marvin Mitchelson, one of California's leading divorce lawyers, reckons that everyone who signs a marriage contract ends up filing for divorce. That way lawyers get a slice of the cake at both ends.

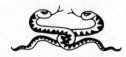

If Dietrich Ekhof of Stuttgart had seen the terms *his* wife had in store for him after their marriage he would have taken to the hills. On their wedding night Dietrich discovered his bride had no intention of allowing him to consummate the marriage until he'd agreed to a set of conditions. The first was that he would hand over his weekly pay packet, unopened, to her. The second, that he would pay the equivalent of £15 every time they made love. The third was that he would never discuss with her his work in the municipal mortuary, because the idea of it upset her. Being a tolerant kind of man, Dietrich agreed to all this and stuck to his side of the bargain until their second child was born, at which time Brigitta doubled the fee for making love. This rise in the cost of loving was too much. Dietrich made an improper advance to one of his wife's young relatives and landed up in court, where his story held the jury spellbound.

'It was very difficult for me,' he explained in his defence. 'I couldn't save enough money to pay her. I asked for credit – but she refused to give me any. In nineteen years I could afford to have her only eighteen times. The strain was terrible.'

When Brigitta was called to give evidence and asked why she imposed such conditions on the marriage, her answer was, 'Nothing in life is free.'

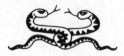

Sylvester Stallone learned that lesson too. A divorce from his first wife Sasha cost him £22,000,000, so when statuesque Brigitte Neilson agreed to wear his wedding ring it was on the strict understanding that hubby paid her £1000 a day, with the promise of a rise if she stuck with him for five years. In return for this £365,000 a year Brigitte agreed to forgo any claims to half of Stallone's property in the event of a divorce.

But the 'salary' was just for starters. On top of that she was promised expenses for clothing, travel and entertainment; over £200,000 for each movie she made with her husband; a cash settlement if they were to divorce and £1,000,000 in trust for each of their children – if the marriage survived long enough to produce any. She was also allowed to keep any gifts Stallone gave her, and in the first four months they included a gold necklace, a fur coat, one dress that cost a cool £7000, a marble dining table with her portrait etched on its surface and a pair of snakeskin boots.

'I feel like Alice in Wonderland. For the first time in my life I'm living like a queen. I can't believe all this money I'm getting – it's like winning a lottery,' she announced, on being questioned about the working agreement. Obviously no one had mentioned Parkinson's Law – expenditure rises to meet income – to her. Rumour had it that after four months of marriage she had already spent the first year's allowance and was asking for an advance on next year's!

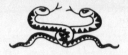

If Jerzy and Kathryn Sluckin had had a pre-marital agreement their marriage might have lasted a little longer than
an hour. Within sixty minutes of leaving Kensington
registry office in November 1975 Kathryn announced to
guests at the reception, 'It won't work,' and disappeared.
Her husband later found her living in a Divine Light
Meditation Commune in Finchley.

'I had a few doubts before the wedding,' she admitted,
'but I didn't want to say anything.'

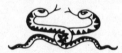

Possibly the *quickest* marriage on record occurred in Nash-
ville in 1974 when Judge Charles Galbreath was
approached by a young couple who asked if the ceremony
could be kept short. 'Do you want to get married?' he
asked them.

'Yes,' they replied.

'You are,' pronounced the judge.

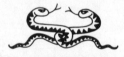

It's not often that weddings turn into funerals, but when
it does happen it's definitely a disaster. In my first book I
recounted the tale of a Pennsylvania couple who were in
the middle of making their vows when the groom col-
lapsed, uttering the binding words 'My God – I do' just as
he expired. On that occasion the wife asked to be declared
an 'official widow'. Now I've found another example
which occurred in China. In China they're not very keen

on kissing as a way of showing affection. What's more, they're not allowed to marry until they're almost into their thirties. Perhaps it was this combination of innocence and lack of practice which led to the demise of a bride in Hunan province when her husband kissed her after the ceremony. Doctors called to the case reported that the passion, intensity and duration of the new husband's kiss on his wife's neck caused heart palpitations that killed her.

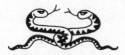

Disasters of a more minor kind frequently occur at weddings. One young soldier, for example, made a note of a hymn he'd particularly enjoyed at a friend's wedding – 'O God of Love, to Thee we Bow' – which was number 774 in the Methodist hymn book. When his own great day came he was still battling with a massive hangover from his stag party and took his pew only a few moments before the bride made her entrance. His late arrival gave the vicar just enough time to whisper, 'Are you sure it's hymn 774 you want?' The soldier answered that he was absolutely certain, and although the vicar still seemed bothered he forgot about it – until, to the congregation's astonishment, they entered into a rousing rendering of:

> Come, O Thou Traveller unknown,
> Whom still I hold, but cannot see,
> My company before is gone,
> And I am left alone with Thee.
> With Thee all night I mean to stay
> And wrestle till the break of day.

How was he supposed to know that instead of the Methodist hymn book they'd be using *Hymns Ancient and Modern*?

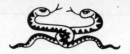

Then there are the occasions when the happy couple escape disaster during the ceremony and begin to relax, thinking they've got away with it. Newlyweds Michael and Donna Dickinson were posing on the lawn of the country hotel in which they were holding their wedding reception while their friends and relatives took pictures. 'Back, back!' cried the amateur photographers, trying to get the couple in focus. Back stepped the couple. 'Back a bit more,' came the instruction. Michael and Donna were so busy staring into each other's eyes they didn't check what was behind them. When they were pulled out of the hotel's ornamental pond they were still holding hands.

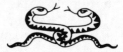

Canadian hot-air balloon enthusiasts Frank and Sue-Lynn Clarke took off from their wedding reception in style. They planned to fly away from the country club in which they'd celebrated with friends and land in a field six miles away, where their car was waiting to take them on honeymoon. Frank and his best man had organized things with great care, but at the last moment there was a change in the wind direction and the balloon carried the newlyweds into a nearby clump of trees. Sue-Lynn escaped unhurt but Frank spent the first six weeks of married life with both arms in plaster.

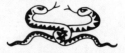

The wedding of Judy and Patrick Crane had to be delayed when a pigeon which had become trapped in the church began frantically dive-bombing the congregation. After some time spent trying to coax the bird out, the vicar called a local farmer who arrived with his gun to dispose of the nuisance. The wedding party were taken to the vicarage for coffee while he did his job. It put rather a damper on the day, according to the bride's mother. Throughout the service the little bridesmaids could be heard sobbing loudly and every now and then a pigeon feather fluttered down from the rafters.

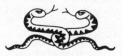

The trouble with being best man at a wedding is that you never get a chance to prove it – or so it was until a wedding held in Galveston, Texas. The bride, twice-married Cindi Friedman, walked down the aisle, stood by the side of her groom, glanced across at the best man – and discovered that he was her first husband. While the clergyman made his introductory remarks the bride and her ex swapped smouldering looks, and by the time it was Cindi's turn to make her responses it was plain to everyone, including the bridegroom, that her heart was no longer in it. There then followed a short interval while the groom and his best man argued and swapped punches. Fortunately one of the guests was a lawyer; he stepped in and it didn't take long to complete the resulting negotiations. Cindi and her newly-intended agreed to pay all the wedding and honeymoon expenses incurred by her jilted lover, plus damages for his emotional and physical pain and suffering. Then the wedding proceeded, this time with the new groom and a new best man.

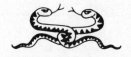

While some people like Cindi Friedman have a surfeit of willing husbands, there are some less fortunate people who have so much trouble proposing that they never make it down the aisle. Here's one example. At the turn of the century a London teacher fell in love with a wealthy Sussex girl called Gwendolin. One weekend he went to stay at the family's ancestral home near Lewes with the intention of proposing to her. During his first night there he woke with a terrible thirst and, reaching for a glass of water in the dark, he knocked something over. At the time he didn't think about it, but daylight revealed that he'd tipped a bottle of ink over a priceless ancient tapestry. He left immediately without popping the question.

Eventually he felt it was safe to go back, though just for a half-hour visit one afternoon. On arrival he asked Gwendolin's mother if he might speak to her daughter and when she went to fetch her sat down on what he thought was a cushion. It was not. It was a Pekingese dog, a favourite with all the family. What was worse, by the time he realized his mistake it was a dead Pekingese dog. He left, never to return, and they both married other people.

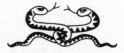

Hank Grove of Cleveland, Ohio, must have been congratulating himself on getting away with a bigamous marriage. Then the first Mrs Grove found uncooked rice in the back of the car and began to wonder exactly what her husband had been catching on all his recent fishing trips . . .

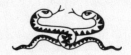

Keith Plummer of Stockport was naturally absent-minded; when he married for the second time he told his new bride all about his first wife – all except for the fact that he wasn't actually divorced from her. When she discovered this the new Mrs Plummer walked out, which spurred Keith into arranging a divorce from wife number one. As it turned out, his first wife had already got there first and divorced him without bothering to let him know. No longer a bigamist, he set out in hot pursuit of his legitimate wife and found that she'd married an old flame on the rebound – thus committing bigamy herself!

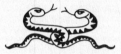

Another husband who sprung a surprise on his wife was Frank Douglas from Newcastle, New South Wales. Hazel Douglas felt that her marriage to him had grown dull and boring, so to try to inject a little fun into her life she placed an anonymous advert that read, 'Sex kitten seeks rampant lion' in a newspaper.

There were a number of replies, including one from her husband who had thoughtfully included a photograph of himself in the nude. That was the first time Hazel had seen him without any clothes on in a dozen years.

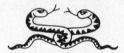

Having an affair can lead to terrible complications, but Janos Istvan found a way of simplifying his love life when he took two girlfriends as well as a wife. Mondays, Wednesdays and Fridays were spent at home in the marriage bed, while Tuesday and Thursday nights were devoted to girlfriend number one and the weekends to girl number two. The problem of getting their names muddled up was solved by asking them all to change their

names to Rosy. When in due course each Rosy gave birth
to a son, he called each baby Stefan. All went as well as
such a complicated arrangement could be expected to go
for four years. Then wife Rosy discovered an address
book containing details of all the other Rosys and Stefans.
She telephoned them, they met, and Janos found himself
in the divorce court and being sued for maintenance by all
three.

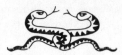

If that sounds complicated, see what you can make of this
Belfast Telegraph report of an incident which led to divorce
proceedings. 'In the divorce action the pursuer, a woman,
apparently masqueraded as another woman and spent the
night with her husband in a hotel in Glasgow. Subse-
quently this other woman started proceedings against her
husband on the grounds of his misconduct with an
unknown woman in the hotel in Glasgow on that
night . . .'

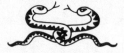

Mrs Mary Lambie, wife of football manager John Lambie,
may well have grounds for divorce following the 1986–7
soccer season. Mr Lambie manages the Scottish Premier
Division team Hamilton Academicals and two matches
into the season he made a vow to remain celibate until his
side won their first match. 'The first time we have a
result, we'll have sex,' he announced to his wife. 'So you
won't have to wait long.' By November he was beginning
to regret those words. Hamilton had failed to achieve a
victory in any of their fifteen Premier Division games and
Mrs Lambie was making sure that he kept to his word.

Although Frenchmen have a reputation for being great lovers, it's not justified if Didier Amboise is anything to go by. Unable to think of anything to do when TV technicians went on strike and blacked out screens all over France, he amused himself by taking pot-shots at his wife. Eventually he hit her and she was taken to hospital. 'There was nothing to watch,' he explained, 'and I was bored.'

From her hospital bed Mme Amboise backed him all the way. 'I don't blame my husband,' she said in her statement. 'It really was very tedious in the evenings.'

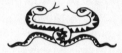

In its proud tradition of eye-catching and racy stories the *News of the World* included this headline in its pages one Sunday morning:

NUDIST WELFARE MAN'S MODEL WIFE FELL FOR THE CHINESE HYPNOTIST FROM THE CO-OP BACON FACTORY.

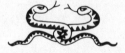

Money can't buy love. If you don't believe it, look at the story of Barbara Hutton, heiress to a forty-five-million-dollar Woolworth fortune. After a number of husbands and countless lovers she set her sights on Porfirio Rubirosa, a Dominican diplomat and internationally renowned lover who was reportedly the model for Harold Robbins's hero in *The Adventurers*. Rubi, as he was known, was celebrated for his conquests, who included Jayne Mansfield, Marilyn Monroe and Evita Peron, and his legendary prowess as a lover. In many chic restaurants at the time diners would ask waiters for 'the Rubirosa' and be brought a sixteen-inch pepper mill!

Rubi wasn't easily won, though. It reputedly cost Barbara Hutton two and a half million dollars before he agreed to make her his wife. She should have known that it wasn't going to work. On the day of the wedding many morning papers carried a picture of Zsa Zsa Gabor, Rubi's most recent girlfriend, sporting a black eye which she said he'd given her because she'd refused to marry him. Undeterred, Barbara went ahead with the ceremony and had her money's worth of Rubi on their wedding night. He, apparently, wasn't as easily satisfied and slipped out of the marital bed to spend the rest of the night with a showgirl. Asked for her comments, Zsa Zsa Gabor gave the marriage six months. It lasted less than three.

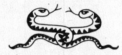

Losing your husband to another woman is a bitter blow for any wife, but when that other woman is your mother it must be particularly hard to bear. When Mrs Jeanette Monk found herself faced with this very situation she gracefully agreed to a divorce and also renounced her custodial rights to her two children. Her ex-husband Alan and her mother, Mrs Valerie Hill, had to apply to the House of Lords for special permission to marry; it was granted and soon Jeanette found that her husband had become her step-father.

The new Mrs Monk, twenty years her husband's senior, knew a thing or two about marriage having had three previous husbands. One she had divorced, the other two had died. To ensure a continuing romance, Alan 'proposed' to her each night and they repeated their marriage vows together daily; perhaps they were as confused as many of their friends had been about their relationship.

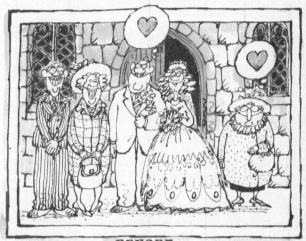

BEFORE

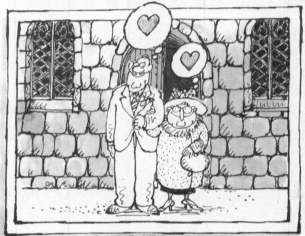

AFTER

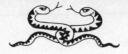

But worse than losing your husband to your mother must be losing him to another man. Even before Nula Ebert married her lawyer husband Leon she had her suspicions that all was not well. She'd once caught him wrestling with another man in the back of a pick-up truck and then on a dinner date he'd disappeared for fifteen minutes with a waiter who'd offered to show him the way to the Gents.

All her fears were borne out on the second day of the honeymoon in Rio when she returned unexpectedly to their hotel room and found Leon enthusiastically humping one of the male guests who'd been at their wedding. Her husband had been so taken with the young man that he'd told him which hotel they would be staying in and provided his air fare. Nula packed her bags and called a divorce lawyer. Leon and his lover spent a fortnight in the honeymoon suite.

All in a
day's work

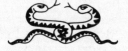

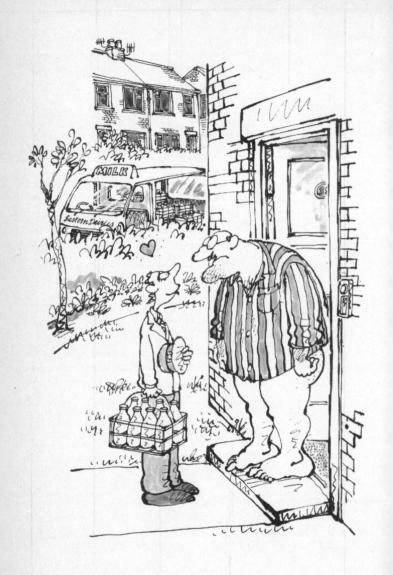

'I don't see Alfred at night any more since he got so interested in sex,' reflected Mrs Alfred Kinsey, whose husband wrote the definitive *Kinsey Report on Sexual Behaviour*. Sociologists like Kinsey, blue movie stars, strippers and ladies of the night are among the more predictable people who make a living from sex. And naturally, where there's sex there's also disaster . . .

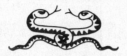

Quite how easily one can fall into the sexual underworld was demonstrated when an American women's magazine did a feature on the blue light districts of a number of European cities. In Copenhagen they interviewed a woman who starred in one of the famous live sex shows. She described how she had sex twelve times a week with a variety of partners and in a number of different routines. And how did she come to have this job? the interviewer wanted to know. The porn star explained that she'd been working as a cleaner at the club when one night the usual girl hadn't turned up; the manager had asked her if *she'd* stand in. Before she knew what was happening she was stark naked and having oral sex with a complete stranger in front of an audience of more than a hundred goggle-eyed punters.

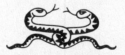

Unemployment is hitting everyone, but milkmen feel particularly robbed. A newspaper survey of on-the-job slap and tickle revealed that milkmen are being deprived of one of the traditional perks of the job. As one explained, 'In the old days – I'm talking about twenty years ago – if a housewife answered the door in her nightie and gave you the come-on you could be certain her old man was at work. These days you ring the doorbell and he comes and pays the milk bill himself.'

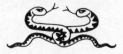

Not so long ago a group of Birmingham councillors came up with the idea of establishing municipal brothels so as to stop soliciting on the streets. The resulting 'rogering on the rates' debate raised a number of issues, not least of which was the question of the union which the ladies would be entitled to join. One suggestion was that they would be eligible to join NALGO, but a letter to *Municipal Engineering* commented, 'Without wishing to start a demarcation dispute, I would suggest that as manual workers their place would be in the National Union of Public Employees.'

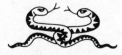

Catering for unusual tastes is something that prostitutes have been doing since the beginning of the oldest profession. One London call-girl found herself entertaining a client whose idea of fun was to make her sit naked on one side of the room with her knees apart while he aimed cream buns at the vital spot. Once out of buns, he covered her breasts with marmalade, decorated her with glacé cherries and proceeded to lick the whole lot off before going away a happy man. Another of her friends had a client with similar tastes. He paid her generously to allow him to play target practice with kippers, which he lobbed across the room in her direction.

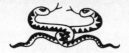

While we're on the subject of milkmen, young Phil Robinson was lucky enough to have a round on which at least half-a-dozen wives had husbands still in work. Before long he was offering all the ladies a very personal kind of service in the mornings. Being a discreet sort of chap, he tried to make sure that none of his regulars got to know about each other – but sadly word soon got around. Most of them didn't mind too much, but one lady was jealous. Phil got back to his float after an energetic bout one morning and discovered that she'd opened every bottle of milk on board and poured the contents in the road.

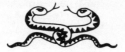

Milkmen are traditionally randy and so are doctors – but at work? An agency nurse on night duty at a Midlands hospital was startled to hear groans coming from one of the curtained-off cubicles in a ward she was supposed to be patrolling. She whipped back the curtains, prepared to find someone in terrible pain, and discovered a young houseman and *two* nurses doing just what the doctor ordered.

Even more shocked was a porter who was asked to take a body down to the mortuary late one night. He wheeled his way in without knocking and surprised two hospital staff who were making love on the mortuary slab.

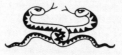

During the making of a very amusing film called *She'll Be Wearing Pink Pajamas* actress Julie Walters and other female

members of the cast were required to appear naked in a
shower scene. They felt that it was unfair that the male
members of the production crew should have a chance to
ogle them, so they decided to get their revenge.

When the director and his crew arrived on set they
found a letter from the actors' union Equity informing
them of a new rule. From now on, the letter explained,
for every actor required to remove his or her clothing on
set, a member of the production team would have to do
likewise. This caused great consternation among the
cameramen and sound recordists and someone was sent to
call the Equity number and check the information. Miss
Walters had anticipated this and arranged for one of her
friends in London to intercept the call and assure the
director that he had to obey the new ruling – which he
did. By the time the actresses admitted it was all a joke
the production crew were out of their clothing and
nervously handling their equipment . . .

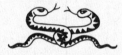

On the film *Caligula* the sex was taken very much more
seriously! When *Penthouse* magazine put up the money for
the movie they envisaged the product as 'a soft-core soft-
focus copy of the magazine'. The director, Tinto Brass,
had other ideas. He wanted to produce 'a kind of anarchist,
hard-core slapstick comedy'. What he actually created was
thousands of feet of such sexually explicit footage that it
took *Penthouse* three years and a string of editors before
they arrived at a final version they felt could be
distributed.

There was no question that Tinto Brass had set about
his task diligently. He threw himself into the auditions.
For some people this part was easy; the man who revealed
that he'd been equipped with not one but two penises
barely had time to do up his flies before his contract was

produced. Many of the actresses had to work harder to prove how convincingly they could convey sexual rapture and more than three hundred of them did screen tests during which they simulated a variety of acts.

When it came to the actual filming, it wasn't all simulation. One orgy took two days to film and many of the participants weren't acting. Tinto Brass was on hand with helpful direction. To one actor, who simply wasn't getting things right, he gave a personal demonstration of oral sex with a Penthouse Pet on set. When Mrs Brass was asked publicly what she thought about this she answered that her husband was only being his usual 'extroverted self'.

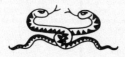

You don't have to be a student of the history of flagellation to know that MPs and members of the legal profession figure largely among the clientele of establishments who specialize in corporal punishment. This year there have been a good number of revelations about spankings and naughty goings-on involving Members of Parliament. For them, of course, it's a personal disaster, but they might take comfort from the reflection that it's nothing new. In fact a hundred years ago Mrs Theresa Berkley of 28 Charlotte Street was the acknowledged expert in such matters.

Her attention to detail was impressive. Her birches were kept permanently in water so that they retained their pliancy. Among her armoury she boasted 'shafts with a dozen whip thongs in them; a dozen different sizes of cat-o'-nine-tails, some with needle points worked into them; various kinds of thin bending canes; leather straps like coach traces; battledores, made of thick sole leather with inch nails run through and curry combs . . .' In season, customers could also look forward to a brisk scourging with fresh nettles.

But the *pièce de résistance* of Mrs Berkley's establishment was her famous Berkley Horse, or Chevalet, a contraption of her own design for flogging customers who were strapped into it so securely that scarcely any part of them could move. Gentlemen travelled from all over Europe to experience this form of perverse pleasure. Among her most fervent fans were a number of MPs. One, in his letter of introduction, wrote that he was 'an ill-behaved young man and quite incorrigible'. His letter went on to spell out his particular requirements and the rewards he offered.

i)   It is necessary that I should be securely fastened to the Chevalet with chains which I will bring myself.
ii) A pound sterling for the first blood drawn.
iii) Two pounds sterling if the blood runs down to my heels.
iv) Three pounds sterling if my heels are bathed in blood.
v)   Four pounds sterling if the blood reaches the floor.
vi) Five pounds sterling if you succeed in making me lose consciousness.

It's nice to know that our current MPs are only upholding traditions from the past!

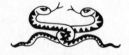

An unexpected hazard of life in the sex business was acknowledged in 1986 when an Old Bailey judge freed a man convicted of an armed robbery at the Windmill Club. John Halsey from Harlow was enticed inside the club and persuaded to order a couple of drinks – orange juice for himself and a glass of 'champagne' (which turned out on inspection to be a soft drink) for a bare-breasted hostess.

The bill for this modest refreshment was £112, which he was forced to pay by a muscular bouncer.

The following week he returned to the club with a replica revolver and an air pistol and forced the two hostesses to hand over the cash box, from which he extracted the money he thought he was owed. When he'd done this he admitted that neither gun was loaded and made an unsuccessful dash for it.

When the case came up in court there was no doubt that most of the people who heard his story were on his side. Even the Crown prosecution admitted that Halsey had 'acted justifiably – if not in method but in motive' and that he had been 'much wronged'. The judge told the two hostesses that he had no sympathy for them and implied that they'd deserved all they'd got, as well as pointing out that in receiving a twelve-month suspended prison sentence instead of immediate jail, Halsey was an exceptional case.

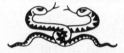

Everyone involved in the business side of sex risks the occasional run-in with the law. In 1966 Copenhagen police decided to raid some of the city's less salubrious sex clubs. In one they interrupted a sixty-six-year-old stripper in the middle of her act. Her stage name was Tuppy and she claimed that she was stripping because her pension wasn't enough to live on.

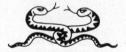

There was panic among New York's high society in 1986 when thirty-two-year-old Sydney Biddle Barrows, who could count George Washington among her forebears, was arrested for running an exclusive call girl racket. The

Catchet, as her organization was known, provided blue-blooded daughters of the republic for blue-chip members of New York's elite.

When it was announced that she might face prosecution for promoting prostitution, an offence that could have put her behind bars for three years, Sydney countered with a warning that in *that* case she would name and subpoena every customer on her books – starting with 340 lawyers. At least three hundred and forty hands immediately began pulling strings on her behalf, and her case was considerably helped when the chief prosecution witness withdrew his evidence after seeing her list of 3500 clients and recognizing the names of the most powerful men in the city.

All the same, justice had to be seen to be done, so Sydney eventually paid a fine amounting to £3000 for a charge so minor it didn't even count as a criminal record against her. New York's elite, saved from the brink of disaster, breathed easy again.

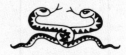

It's not possible to insure against most sexual disasters but blue movie actor Garard Damiano, who took the lead in *Deep Throat*, arranged an insurance policy which covered him against any paternity claims as a result of his work. And Wili Bausch, a West German porn actor, tried to insure his ten-inch organ against accidental damage. However, when the insurance company checked out the nature of his work which in the past had included scenes of (fake) castration, torture and bondage they decided he wasn't a good risk.

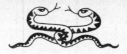

When chauffeur Charles Robinson invested in a £75,000, 24-foot stretch limousine complete with cocktail cabinet, stereo-stack system, radar detector, sound-proofing, CB radio, video and optional double bed he quite expected some of his guests to enjoy a little hanky-panky while he drove them around London and its environs. Among his customers were the rich and famous, and business seemed to be booming; then Charles announced he was selling the car.

Some of his clients had ordered him to kerb-crawl through London while they looked for a girl to tumble in the back. Others brought along their own hard-core movies for entertainment. For one orgy a weary Charles had to keep driving all night. 'Some of these people are not all they seem to be on stage or television,' he admitted when he traded in his passion wagon. 'We've been shocked and disappointed.'

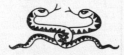

A male stripper had to be rescued by police after he ventured too close to the all-female audience in a Manhattan club and disappeared under a scrum of flailing limbs. The club's management explained that the two bouncers who normally enforced a 'look, don't touch' policy were busy elsewhere when the incident occurred. Unable to restore order, and worried about the safety of the stripper, known as Damien, they called the cops. They were quite right to worry about him, too. By the time he was rescued from under a thirty-nine-year-old secretary who was bouncing astride him, he was unconscious. And the doctor

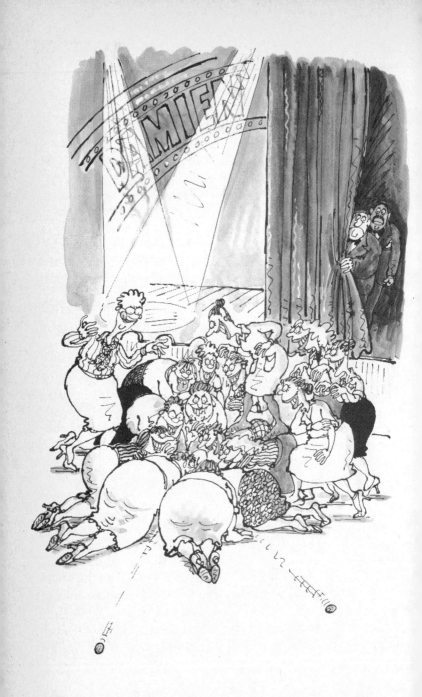

who admitted him to hospital said it looked as if someone had been trying to twist his balls off.

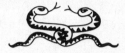

Someone else who was screwed in the course of his work was a Bordeaux tax inspector who decided to investigate the financial affairs of the city's prostitutes. The first he visited admitted that she hadn't made a tax return in her life. Instead of prosecuting, the taxman offered to forget the offence in return for sexual favours. He came to similar arrangements with a number of other prostitutes until he tried his line with one who really *did* pay income tax. She reported him to his boss and the sex-mad civil servant was taken to court where he admitted blackmailing no fewer than seventy-five women.

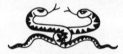

Hedwige Kiesler, daughter of a merchant banker, found herself in the blue movie business because she didn't read her contract. Hedy Lamarr, as she later became known, was a star-struck beauty of sixteen when in 1929 she was offered the part of a water nymph; she signed without checking the small print and cursed her stupidity for the rest of her career.

The outline of the film which she'd been shown gave her just a vague idea of her part. Only when it was too late to pull out did she discover that she was required to play several scenes naked; when she protested, the producer pointed out the paragraph in her contract which stated that if she dropped out of the film she would be required to refund the whole cost. She tried to reach a compromise, and as a result the outdoor scenes were shot at a respectable distance, but in the studio where the naked sex scenes were filmed the director would stand just out of camera shot and prick her bare bottom with a pin if he wanted a bit more passion from his leading lady.

By the time the film, *Ecstasy*, was shown, young Hedwige had met and married millionaire Fritz Mandl. The movie's première caused a sensation in Vienna and Fritz was understandably upset to see his gorgeous young wife bared for public view. He immediately locked her away under guard while he tried to buy up every print of the film he could find. The film's producers had a field day; the more prints they made from the negative, which they were careful to keep safe, the more money they coined. While Fritz was wasting his money his wife made a bolt for freedom, headed for America and met a man called Louis B. Mayer, who knew a star when he saw one. She never looked back. Meanwhile poor Fritz was left with a stack of films to remind him of what he was missing, and a huge hole in his bank account.

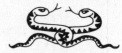

Some people will do anything to get a job. Not so long ago a man exposed himself to a woman working at the Ipswich office of the Department of Health and Social Security because he thought it might help him get work.

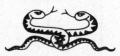

Stunning London University student Gillian Goodman was sorely tempted when someone she knew offered her £1000 to appear in a blue movie he was making. Gillian weighed up the disadvantages, most notably what her boyfriend, fellow student Steve Hutchings, would say if he knew, and then said yes. On the Saturday she was due to make her movie appearance she kissed goodbye to

Steve, who was setting off for a canoeing trip, then nervously went to St John's Wood where the film was being made.

The director ran through the script with her, then suggested she remove her clothing so that they could begin filming. She was stark naked when her co-star arrived. You guessed it. It was Steve.

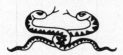

For most people in the sex business it's quite a compliment to be considered indecent – it proves you're doing things properly. That's why stripper Melinda Safian wasn't too pleased when she was acquitted of a charge of indecency in 1985. Although Detective Ron Ziolkowski of the Toledo vice squad had arrested her, he admitted in court that her stage act had not aroused him. The judge concluded that if her act hadn't caused lustful thought or desire in the watchful detective, it couldn't be deemed obscene. After the verdict Ms Safian said worriedly, 'I'm not sure whether I gained or not.'

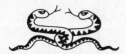

Mavisa Lonez doesn't have to worry about *her* act. It's indecent – and that's official. When she appeared in court in San Fernando, Chile, the judge asked her to demonstrate the exotic dancing that had landed her in trouble. She swung into action with a performance so thrilling that when it came to an end the jury jumped up and gave her a big round of applause. Once the cheers died down they delivered a verdict of guilty and she was fined £25.

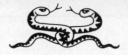

Definitely not indecent was the pornographic material offered by a Swiss bookseller in 1970. Those lusty residents of Biel who succumbed to his advertisements claimed that they'd expected something sexually erotic in the books and not the close-ups of curtains, cushions and household items that tastefully obscured the most interesting bits of the pictures. The would-be pornographer was fined the equivalent of £45 and given a ten-month suspended jail sentence – to teach him to be obscene, we presume.

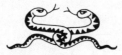

One anonymous Kissagram girl has a very noble view of her work, as she described it to magistrates in Devizes. 'I'm an ambassador of fun,' she explained. 'It's my job to spread laughter and happiness wherever I go.' Her employer agreed, though he did admit that on this occasion the girl, whose speciality was 'Boobagrams', had gone a bit far.

That was something of an understatement. Having arrived at a firm of accountants dressed in corset, stockings and suspenders, she had proceeded to tear off all her clothes while singing 'Happy Birthday to You' to a bemused member of staff. According to one account she then rubbed her breasts provocatively over his body before unzipping his trousers, removing his underpants and pinning him to a desk, apparently with the intention of clambering on top of him. Unfortunately the object of her desire was deeply shocked by the experience and failed to show signs of arousal. Even more unfortunately, she soon realized that she had called at the wrong firm.

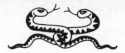

An Ohio lady had lots of misgivings about going to a neighbour's party where she knew blue movies would be shown, but she went – and was glad she had, for in one movie she spotted her husband. 'He was wearing a mask over his face, but I knew it was him all the same,' she told a divorce court. 'He has a birthmark on one buttock, and we saw a lot of it during the film.' She also recalled that it now made sense of a time two years before when he'd come home and wanted to make love to her – with a paper bag over his head.

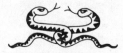

In court for traffic offences was seventy-seven-year-old Cardiff pensioner David Philips, who was fined £5 in 1975 for stealing kisses from forty-two traffic wardens. His motive must have been the uniform – and to many men a severe uniform is terribly sexy. *So* sexy that after several approaches one lovely London traffic warden decided that she could earn more on her back than pounding the pavements on her feet. She was eventually caught in the act by another warden who stuck a ticket on the wind-screen of an illegally parked lorry and then heard suspicious noises coming from the back . . .

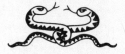

Designer Helen Crowther was caught out from behind too. She was enjoying a fling with a fellow designer at the studio where she worked and had managed to keep it a secret from her regular boyfriend for some time. Then one day she got home from work, stripped off in front of him, and the secret was out. Stuck firmly to her derrière with Cow Gum, the special adhesive designers use, were three little bits of paper that had last been seen on her lover's desk. He'd been about to stick them on a piece of work when Helen had taken him by surprise!

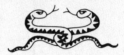

Someone who also had sex on the job was Meg Wallis, a Philadelphia cleaning lady whose sunny smile cheered the elderly people she worked with at two sheltered housing projects. It was only after five of the male residents of the homes, with an average age of seventy-one, went down with VD that anyone realized that it was more than her smile which Mrs Wallis was spreading around. She was immediately fired, at which the gentlemen she had been secretly pleasuring rebelled, protesting that she was the best thing that had happened to them for years. Mrs Wallis was reinstated, but only after everyone involved had had a course of medical treatment.

Evening,
officer . . .

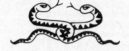

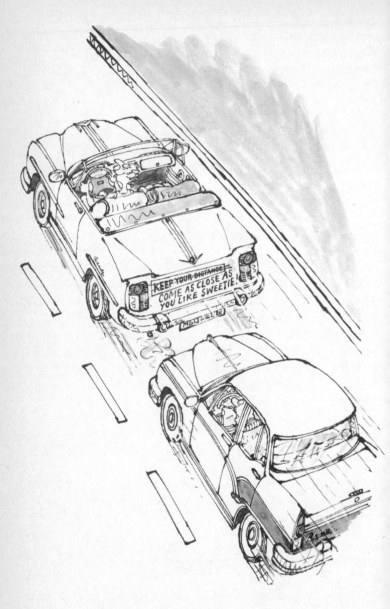

A rare sexual disaster (See page 134)

'It ain't no sin if you crack a few laws now and then, just so long as you don't break any,' said law-abiding Mae West. She knew that when it comes to having a really good time, sex and the law aren't always completely compatible . . .

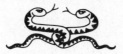

A police patrol car which had followed a Mini Metro being driven erratically through narrow lanes near Grassington, Yorkshire, was just about to overtake and stop the driver when he ran into a stone wall. The policemen pulled open the door and found not one person in the Metro's driving seat but two – a man facing in the correct direction and astride him a young woman, facing the rear window and with her clothing in disarray. From their flushed faces and breathless attitude the police concluded that the crash had coincided with the driver's climax.

In court later the young lady disputed the evidence provided by the police. She and her driving instructor, for that was who he was, had been having a driving lesson and he was taking her home, she explained. Because she had a dry throat she had been reaching across the car from her position in the passenger seat to find the Polo mints that her friend kept in his right-hand trouser pocket. The impact of the crash had thrown her into his lap. When asked why she had removed her underwear and hitched up her skirt before reaching for the Polos she replied that she was a nudist and believed in getting as much fresh air to the body as possible.

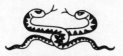

It's not just lawbreakers who find themselves in trouble. A Californian judge had to be removed from office

because he would insist on using a plastic dildo instead of
the more usual gavel to bash the bench for silence.

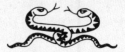

On their return from honeymoon newlyweds David and
Leslie Patterson moved into their neat terraced house in
Coventry. Next door lived a quiet middle-aged bachelor.
For the first few months David and Leslie spent their free
daylight hours decorating and renovating the house and
the rest of the time making enthusiastic love. Then winter
came and with it the need to insulate the loft. This was
the first time David had been up in the roof and above
their bedroom ceiling he found a love bug – a baby alarm
which had been positioned to monitor their most intimate
frolics. The police were called and followed the wire
through the party wall and down to the speakers in their
neighbour's hi-fi system. He tried explaining in court that
he'd only installed the device as a burglar alarm. The
judge was not impressed.

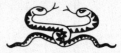

The long, hot summer of 1976 released the British from a
lot of their inhibitions. In Sutton Park, Warwickshire,
police had to be called in to clamp down on the activities
of a group of young girls who had taken to late-night
nude swimming parties. Their naked cavorting was
embarrassing courting couples.

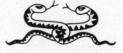

Late one night the emergency line to the police headquar-
ters in Seattle buzzed into life and the duty officer lifted

the receiver to hear what sounded like a violent attack in progress. Within seconds the call had been traced and a patrol car was racing to the scene. Outside the house officers saw a light on in the living room and without wasting time, smashed straight through the window to rescue the victim. They found her writhing ecstatically beneath her boyfriend and the telephone receiver lying on the floor.

Just to prove that their mission hadn't been in vain the officers booked the lovers for improper use of the emergency services. When they appeared in court both pleaded that the call could have been made by accident when they'd got carried away. 'I guess I could have pushed the buttons with my feet,' admitted a blushing Lindy Chapman. The case was dismissed but the lovers were warned to be more careful where they enjoyed themselves in future.

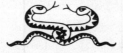

Portsmouth police arrested a couple at the city's station after they'd tried to sell pornographic pictures to passers-by. The pictures weren't much good and they were also rather small, but in the circumstances they showed initiative.

When questioned by detectives the couple admitted that they had met only twenty minutes before their arrest. Both were short of money for their train fare so they'd nipped into the station's photo booth and posed for some dirty pictures that they hoped would raise the extra cash they needed.

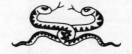

If Lesley Wallace had been a Boy Scout he might have been better prepared for the first night of his honeymoon. As it was, instead of enjoying himself in the arms of his new wife he found himself down at Eastbourne police station charged with breaking into a contraceptive vending machine. As he told the magistrate when his case came up, his wife had refused to let him into bed until he was suitably equipped. Then they found that neither of them had any change!

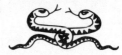

A forty-eight-year-old Neapolitan housewife was enjoying a lie-in one morning after her husband had set off for work when a total stranger burst into the room and climbed into bed with her. Guiseppi Miele, aged twenty-five, had earlier that morning been caught stealing a van full of dishwashers by the police. He'd ditched the vehicle and made a run for it – straight through Signora Giovanna Cifuni's bedroom door. At the time the signora did not appreciate his company. She kicked him out of bed and beat him so violently with a broomstick that he staggered into the street and threw himself at the feet of a policeman begging protection.

Later, when she'd had time to think things over, the signora admitted, 'I must confess that although I kicked up such a fuss I was rather flattered.'

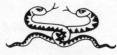

A group of suspected bank raiders appeared in a Genoa court not so long ago and during the trial witnesses were called to identify them. All were certain about the male suspects but there was some doubt about the girl in the gang. She had been wearing a mask during the raid and the only thing that the witnesses could agree on was that she'd been extremely well-developed. The judge pondered for a minute, then asked the girl in the dock if she would lift her jumper so that they could form an unbiased opinion themselves. After a quick word with her lawyer she agreed. The court declared her innocence and she was immediately set free.

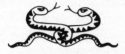

When Pierre Gervais from Mont Laurier, Quebec, lost his girlfriend to a law student he went out and stole a car with the intention of killing himself. The car broke down before he'd had a chance to do so, and he stole another. This one he crashed into a tree, but it was so slow that it barely put a dent in the bumper. While he was sitting behind the wheel wondering what to do next the Mounties drove up and booked him for taking the car and driving it away. While they filled out the paperwork he grabbed one of their pistols, turned the gun on himself and fired – shooting himself in the leg. After a fortnight in hospital he made a brief court appearance and was sentenced to two years in prison. Still suicidal, while he was being escorted to his cell he broke away from his escort and plunged twenty feet through a window. A snowdrift broke his fall.

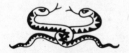

Another failed suicide appeared in court in Stoke-on-Trent. The man claimed that he'd decided to end it all following a row with his girlfriend. The prosecution challenged this assertion, saying that if the man had been seriously set on suicide he wouldn't have thrown himself under a stationary car.

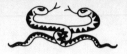

When police in Los Angeles arrested Hal Lockwood for standing naked on a street corner they never reckoned on his being acquitted for lack of evidence. But with no available independent witness that was just what happened. Hal could hardly believe his luck and to celebrate promptly dropped his trousers and exposed himself in the courtroom lobby. He wasn't so lucky a second time round when the same officers booked him for indecent exposure. His plea that he was only 'expressing his joy' was countered by more than enough witnesses.

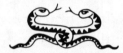

A typographical error in the *Crawley Observer* gave a more graphic description of a local crime than was perhaps intended! 'A man indecently exposed himself to a twelve-year-old girl in Grattons Park, Pound Hill, on Tuesday evening last week. Police said he was about forty with a black beard and short curly black hair, and short curly black hair.'

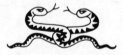

A would-be rapist broke into a women's dormitory block on a university campus in the American mid-west. Bursting into one student's room he announced what he intended to do. Then things began to go wrong. Instead of becoming hysterical and begging him not to, the girl, who was majoring in psychotherapy, began to talk him out of the attack. She was a lesbian, she explained.

This prompted an admission from the rapist that he was

homosexual himself. The student was very understanding and said she knew that one of the night porters at the dorm was gay and that he might appreciate the man's attention. Her argument seemed logical, so the man abandoned his attempt at rape, thanked his 'victim' and went in search of the porter. When he appeared in court he was found guilty of attempted sodomy, sexual abuse and attempted robbery. The jury found him guilty of all three.

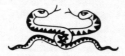

A rape victim of a different sort was eighty-seven-year-old Frank Murray of Altoona, Pennsylvania, who served five years of a life sentence for rape. Then new evidence was produced and a federal judge accepted the argument that Murray could not have been guilty of the offence since he was eighty-two at the time of the alleged assault, almost completely blind, and crippled with arthritis.

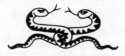

Still on the matter of rape, British judges who are accused of being too lenient when it comes to sentencing rapists might take a lesson from a judge in Arkansas who sentenced a sex offender in his court to 1500 years. When the defence attorney questioned whether this wasn't a bit over the top, even for the crime of rape, the judge answered that it was a reasonable sentence and added that, 'five hundred years would have been just a slap on the wrist.'

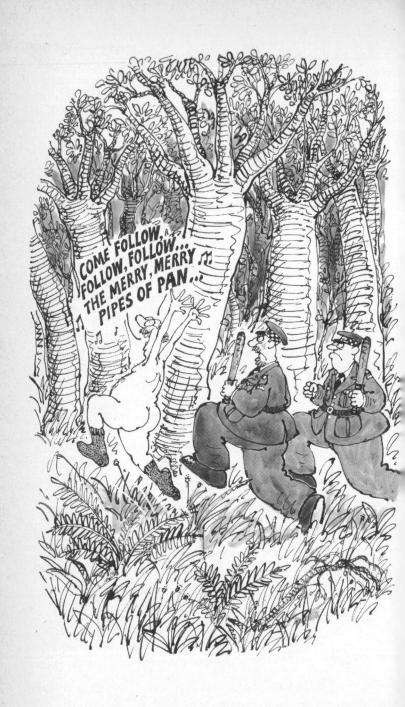

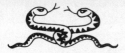

A man brought before a Sheriff in Strathclyde after being apprehended dancing naked in a wood tried pleading that he had been answering the primeval call of the pagan deity of flocks and herds. The Sheriff told him that the great god Pan had not been in the habit of wearing socks.

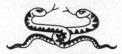

During the trial of one sex offender Mr Mervyn Griffith-Jones, prosecuting counsel, opposed an application for bail made by the defendant. He told the judge, 'It is a perfectly ordinary little case of a man charged with indecency with four or five guardsmen . . . '

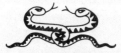

Also the cause of some amusement in court was a man whose domestic problems were summed up in the *Western Daily Press*. 'A man who has made five authenticated suicide attempts, who is separated from a wife he married knowing she was pregnant by another man, who is the father of two children by different women, who is about to become a father by yet another woman, and who admits that he is homosexual cannot be regarded as entirely normal.'

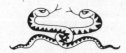

In the spring of 1986 a French court was astonished at the 'not entirely normal' revelations that resulted from the case of a former diplomat and his Chinese mistress who stood in the dock accused of passing secrets to the Chinese. It would be impossible to imagine a more bizarre case. Bernard Boursicot, the diplomat, had been serving in one of France's more out-of-the-way embassies; in Ulan Bator, to be precise. Among the precious secrets passed to the Chinese were such vital observations as, 'One comes across a lot of yaks in this country.'

But even more outrageous were the details of his mistress. To put it bluntly, she was no lady. Despite being a favourite of Mao Tse Tung and a star of the Chinese opera, where she was famed for her sex appeal, Shi Pei Pu was – a man. The judge simply couldn't believe that Boursicot didn't know the secrets of his 'mistress' after a twenty-year relationship. 'Do you mean that you, a Frenchman, are incapable of telling the difference between a man and a woman?' he asked. Obviously this revelation came as a blow to national pride.

The wretched diplomat had to admit that he hadn't known anything was wrong. Shi Pei Pu had even borne him a child – although he had been away on another posting at the time. The child, Shi Du Du, appeared in court, where it was revealed that blood tests proved him not to be Boursicot's son. His 'mother' admitted that she had bought him as an orphan in a street market and pretended that he was Boursicot's boy so that her spying mission could continue. At the end of the whole sorry saga, which entertained the nation for weeks, the disgraced diplomat and his extraordinary lover were both jailed for six years.

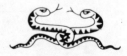

Police were called to an East Sussex church fête after the Brownies, who had just performed a selection of traditional country dances on the vicarage lawn, skipped back to the Brownie hut and surprised a couple who were hard at it. Waiting their turn at the rear door of the hut were three other men with five-pound notes. 'I was driving through Hastings when God spoke and told me to give myself to the church,' the woman explained when her case came up in court. The magistrate said that he doubted whether God had meant it quite like that, and taking her previous record for prostitution into account he fined her £50.

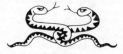

A Prestwick man whose idea of a bit of rough and tumble was to be jumped on, walked on and kicked by a couple of girls, found himself in court after offering the pair £1 each to abuse him in this way. Giving evidence, the girls described how the man had approached them in the street with this suggestion. Both were asked to identify the defendant when they stepped into the dock. One girl did this successfully, but the other picked out the court's official shorthand recorder before being asked by the Procurator-Fiscal to take a more thorough look round.

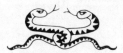

Down in Fort Lauderdale, Florida, they were getting worried about the rapidly rising tide of pornography sweeping through America. To combat this the City Commission passed a draconian by-law banning all obscenity in magazines, books and records. Then it was discovered that the stringencies of the new law extended to its very own wording – which meant that it couldn't be published.

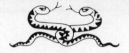

Marvin Hunter, a twenty-five-year-old delivery man from Springfield, Ohio, was the victim of a rare sexual disaster when a truck ran into the rear of his delivery van and turned Marvin into a homosexual.

Physically he suffered only minor injuries to his back but, as he pleaded in court, the prang had had a catastrophic effect on his personality and radically altered his sexual urges. He left his wife, started to frequent gay bars and, once lured into gay literature, knew there was no turning back. The jury awarded a quarter of a million dollars in compensation – and gave Mrs Hunter $25,000 in lieu of what she'd lost.

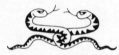

Raymond Duchene became the victim of a sexual disaster without even having sex. He was called as a witness during a trial in which one of his associates stated that Duchene had committed adultery with his wife. This Duchene admitted, even going so far as to describe the encounter in torrid detail. The lady with whom he was supposed to have made love denied every word of it and challenged him to describe her tummy button. At this point he was caught out; not having had the pleasure of her, he wasn't aware that she had an artificial navel that had been sculpted by a plastic surgeon. It was the tummy button that cost him his freedom, for he was charged on a count of perjury.

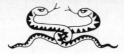

It was shyness that made Mark Currie turn to crime. When he was caught breaking into a Midlands sex shop in the early hours of the morning he confessed that his only reason for committing the crime was that he was too embarrassed to go into the place when there were other people around.

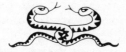

In 1987 Brisbane waiter Barry Tadday appeared in court charged with slapping a girl's bottom as she walked past him – seventeen years after he'd done the deed. Both he and his victim had forgotten all about it, but the authorities were determined to get their man. When he applied for a taxi driver's licence and police files were routinely searched, they came up with a warrant for his arrest. Fortunately the judge had a sense of proportion. Despite the fact that Tadday pleaded guilty he quashed the charge.

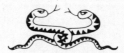

Another man whose past caught up with him was shop assistant Michael O'Connor who was taken to court for kissing a customer in 1907. He explained that he'd been in high spirits because it was such a lovely day, but he was jailed nevertheless. Ten years later he received a solicitor's letter. The woman he'd so impulsively embraced, Miss Hazel Moore, had died and left him £20,000 in her will in memory of the only time in her life she'd been kissed by a man.

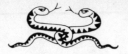

I don't suppose many of the players objected when well-endowed Morgana Roberts, a topless go-go dancer from Houston, Texas, invaded the pitch during a game. The police didn't approve, though, and she was arrested. In court her lawyer explained that Ms Roberts, whose bust measures an amazing sixty inches, was merely leaning on a rail and watching the game when she overbalanced and toppled on to the pitch. Her court appearance didn't seem to bother her. While she waited for the verdict she signed autographs and joked with goggle-eyed officials.

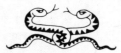

Two weeks after starting her job as a double-glazing salesperson, calling on people in their own homes, Debbie Hartley's order books were bulging. Fellow salespeople wondered what she did to persuade so many customers to buy. They found out when the police were called by a man alleging that she had behaved indecently in his lounge. Investigations revealed that her selling technique involved wearing a low-cut blouse with no bra, and promising to remove the garment if a male customer signed on the dotted line.

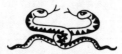

Vanna Henrikson couldn't have found a worse day to begin her life as a prostitute if she'd tried. Ten minutes after she walked nervously into the bar of a hotel in Geneva she was on her way to the police station. She wasn't to know that the hotel was hosting an international conference on vice and that almost every man in the place was a police chief, was she?

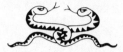

Two daredevil German tourists who went paragliding over Palma Bay in Majorca surprised onlookers by dropping their bathing costumes once they were airborne and getting stuck in. The man steering the boat was alerted by the cheering crowds at the edge of the water and cut the line that linked the parachute to his craft. The naughty Germans swam to a raft where they stayed, despite police attempts to call them in. Eventually the police gave up and went home and the cheeky couple were able to return to dry land.

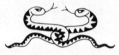

When asked by Cambridgeshire police how she had recognized the man who had jumped, naked, out of a bush as she was crossing a park late one night, the flasher's victim said that she was familiar with his equipment. His equipment? questioned the detective. Which part of his equipment precisely? His Ronald Reagan face mask? His training shoes? His *anatomy*? None of those, said the witness. It was his bicycle lamp, with which he had illuminated the part of his anatomy he was most proud of, that had given him away. It was held together by a distinctive piece of yellow sticky tape, which she herself had applied when her boss had dropped his bike lamp in the office . . .

A Clapham flasher had both the police *and* ambulance services out when he rang a doorbell and then pushed his penis through the letterbox, presumably in an attempt to impress the woman who had just let herself into the house. She was not amused and snapped the letterbox flap down on the offending part of his anatomy. When the screams from outside subsided both she and the flasher realised that he was stuck. It took twenty minutes to free him, by which time the police had taken down all his particulars.

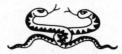

When police raided a pornographic bookshop in Hamburg they removed several thousands of pounds worth of obscene publications which were to provide evidence at the subsequent trial. Unfortunately when the time came for the trial the books, held in secure police custody, had mysteriously disappeared. Perhaps it shouldn't come as too much of a surprise. After all, when a Canadian vice-squad team raided a sex store they suspected of selling obscene material they found one of their own officers already there – as a customer.

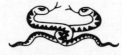

A stunning topless French girl and a man taking photos of her as she posed in Trent Park, Cockfosters (yes, *really!*), were arrested after park staff alerted police. The girl tearfully explained that the man had told her he was a film director and wanted to do some test shots to see if she was photogenic. She was allowed to go after they'd told her that he had no film in his camera.

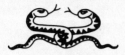

Finally, an anonymous mounted policewoman brought a heckler down to size during the miners' strike after he'd observed, 'Hey, love, your horse is foaming at the mouth.'

'I'm not surprised,' commented the implacable law lady. 'So would you be if you'd been between my legs for the last two hours.'

Surprise, surprise!

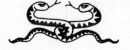

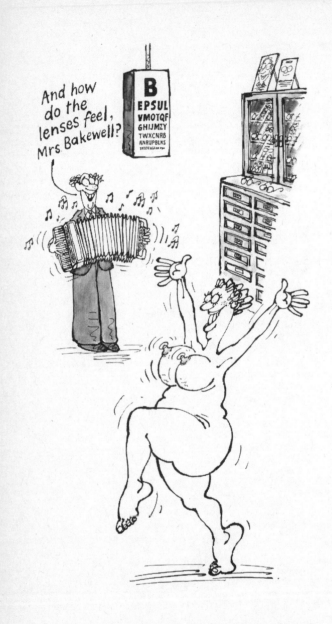

'Boy, am I exhausted! I went on a double date last night and the other girl didn't show up,' said Mae West after what must have been a pleasant surprise. Other sexual tricks and hoaxes are distinctly more disastrous . . .

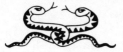

Turin ladies who went to see psychiatrist Alfredo Buscoli felt greatly relaxed after a session on the couch with him, for Alfredo had a therapy not on offer elsewhere. His habit was to slip his female patients drugs to send them to sleep, then to strip them naked and photograph them in a variety of revealing poses. When the police caught up with him and discovered a suitcase full of naughty negatives Alfredo explained, 'I showed the pictures to my patients to help free them from their inhibitions . . .'

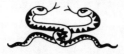

Another story with medical overtones was reported in Holland in 1979 when an optician was charged with various offences relating to his female patients. It was alleged that when women visited his consulting room they were told to remove their clothes and dance while he played the accordion. 'This test was carried out to make sure they were the right kind for contact lenses,' the optician's lawyer explained.

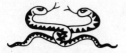

The man who persuaded his lady passenger to take off her bra so that he could use it as a fanbelt must have been pretty persuasive. Also gifted with the powers of persuasion was a rabbi who gave spiritual help to thirty-two-year-old Sipora Keltzerman. She suffered from a skin ailment that was proving difficult to cure. The rabbi offered spirit healing and told her that her only chance of a cure was to take off her clothes, lie down and make love to him. 'It's not for my pleasure, you understand,' he told her. 'It is to please the angels that will heal you . . . ' Oh *really*?

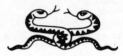

Most of us have stories to tell about honeymoon japes – confetti stuffed into the pockets of going-away outfits, ancient kippers hidden inside the car, booby-trapped beds and so on – but few could hope to rival that of Dr Simon Wheaton. He passed out while celebrating his stag night with other members of the hospital rugby team and came to with his leg in plaster up to his thigh. He'd slipped and broken it, his friends told him; if he hadn't been so drunk it could have been a lot worse. Simon put on a brave face and hobbled through the wedding – and through the honeymoon too. It was only when he and his long-suffering wife got back that his friends revealed that his leg had never been broken. If he hadn't been so smashed he would never have been plastered.

Colin Entwhistle was invited to a wedding on 20 July 1985. He turned up, wearing his best suit, but couldn't find his girlfriend Julie among the guests at the front of the registry office. 'Go inside,' suggested someone. He did, and by the time he came out he was a married man.

'We've been trying to get married for ages,' bubbled Julie, having got her man at last, 'so I thought I'd give him a surprise and get everything organized. He looked a bit nervous when he finally realized it was his own wedding but he didn't make any fuss. He's been a bit quiet but he'll get over it.' Colin just smiled wanly.

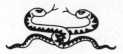

Not long after her wedding a New Jersey woman answered a telephone call from a man who said he was her husband's sex therapist. He wanted her to help with her husband's treatment, he explained, and she agreed to do so – even when he told her to stop what she was doing, go outside and have sex with the first man she met. The lucky chap happened to be her next-door neighbour, who agreed to help her out.

When her husband got home that evening his wife assured him that she was willing to do *anything* to help his sexual problem. This comforting support didn't have the desired effect, because the husband protested that he'd never been to a sex therapist in his life. He had to be restrained from going next door to murder his neighbour.

When the police were called they put a tap on the telephone line and before the week was out had traced a second call to the vice-president of the company that owns the world-famous Harlem Globetrotters basketball team. He was charged with sexual harassment.

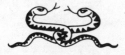

The editor of *Cosmopolitan* magazine had a surprise when she met Jane White, runner-up in the magazine's New Journalist of the Year competition in 1986. As we all know, the quintessential Cosmo woman is intelligent, witty, informed and feminine. It was these qualities that shone with such impact from Jane White's pieces on pre-marital terror and today's ideal man. The impact was not diminished when editor Linda Kelsey met the writer at the prize-giving and Jane White turned out to be a Liverpool van driver called Kevin Sampson.

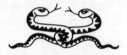

After a fall from a ladder a Bristol bricklayer was admitted to the accident and emergency department of the local hospital. There, despite his discomfort, he so enjoyed having his clothes removed by the nurses that he returned on several occasions pretending to be unconscious in the hope that it would happen again. One female doctor who encountered him and couldn't tell if he was really unconscious or not decided to call his bluff. She and a nurse stripped off his jeans and Y-fronts, then gave him a blast of icy local anaesthetic around the balls. The patient leapt to his feet and tugged on his underwear before racing off. He never bothered them again.

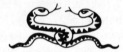

A medical hoaxer of a different kind struck in 1985 when a man set up a practice in south London. He called himself a doctor, but it didn't take long for his patients to suss that he was up to no good. As one young lady pointed out, 'I got very suspicious when I went in complaining of a sore throat and he said he'd have to do an internal examination. At first I thought he meant my throat – but he didn't. He said it was all to do with antibodies but I didn't believe him.'

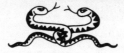

Many men fantasize about the kind of liberties they could take as doctors. The youngest hoaxer of this kind on record was a sixteen-year-old boy who stole the school doctor's stethoscope, borrowed his father's car and took off in the direction of the local girls' school in a white coat. Once there he persuaded the school's matron to provide him with the facilities to examine young girls. He might have got away with it, too, if after a morning's happy inspection one of the girls hadn't recognized him.

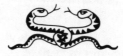

When the news of a Sex Olympics was announced in 1971 it caused instant excitement. The *News of the World* thrilled at the concept and headlined it as 'the most shocking sporting event ever to be screened', and reporters eagerly volunteered to cover the action. Meanwhile the promoter, Dr Harrison Rogers, gave a news briefing outlining the features of this truly international event. Several countries had already agreed to field teams, he announced, and the judging would be undertaken by a panel of respected authorities including doctors and psychologists. He also promised that the press would receive invitations as soon as the qualifying heats had been organized.

It was standing room only when the invitations finally arrived. Dr Rogers and a beautiful blonde introduced a series of filmed excerpts from the first rounds of the heats. The journalists watched intently; the film clips were enough to steam up anyone's glasses. But the mist soon cleared when the lights went up and Dr Rogers peeled off his beard and told the startled company that he'd been pulling their legs just a little. His real name was Alan

Abel, a notorious practical joker, and he went on to explain that what they'd been watching were some rushes from his blue movie parody. He hadn't got much cash left for publicity so he'd invented the Sexual Olympics as a way of attracting attention – and boy had he got it!

Another con man orchestrated the uproar that hit New York in 1917. Anthony Comstock, president of New York City's Anti-Vice League, was a tireless champion of the pure and good. He was absolutely guaranteed to spot anything salacious and make a fuss about it – so when he heard that a group of young Brooklyn boys had been seen clustering outside a shop that displayed in its window a picture of a naked woman, things began to happen. He demanded that the shopkeeper remove the picture; the shopkeeper refused. The court case that followed attracted national attention and the offending picture was spread across the front pages from coast to coast. Preachers spoke against its evil in church; music-hall entertainers mentioned it in their acts – which was exactly what a press agent called Harry Reichenberg wanted.

The picture involved in the fuss was called 'September Morn' by French artist Paul Chabas. It showed a naked but demure maiden standing beside the sea in the morning mist. An advertising agent for a Brooklyn brewery had spotted it and ordered 2000 copies to decorate the firm's 1917 calendar. These had been printed and delivered before someone higher up decided that the picture was not suitable. The job-lot of 2000 pictures had been snapped up by a shopkeeper who then found he couldn't sell them. Which was where Reichenberg came in. He'd paid the crowd of urchins to goggle at the picture in the window and he'd helped to orchestrate the outcry, relying on Comstock's blustering self-righteousness to do the rest of the work for him. By the time the court case was in full swing those 2000 pictures that no one had wanted were worth their weight in gold.

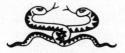

The New York publishing world pricked up its ears when news of a new book, *I, Libertine*, began to circulate. The book was the life story of an eighteenth-century rake, researched and written by a retired naval officer who had made a special study of the period's pornography and erotica. It promised to have all the ingredients of a best-seller – plenty of explicit sex but in a 'respectable' form.

News of the title first broke in the *New York Times* when it was listed among forthcoming titles. A number of literary periodicals ran features on the author. Book reviewers started receiving calls from editors wondering why they hadn't read it. And a student at Cornell University even wrote a dissertation on the novel and its historical background and was awarded a respectable mark for it. Everyone waited in anticipation for publication day – and went on waiting, because in reality *I, Libertine* had never existed outside the imagination of an all-night disc jockey called Gene Shepard and his small band of insomniac listeners. The whole thing was a hoax. Such was the level of interest, though, that a publisher suggested to Shepard that he write the book for real. When it appeared it almost lived up to the pre-publicity of the spoof!

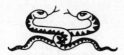

Mike McGrady's surprise was in the field of publishing too. Looking along the lines of popular paperbacks in his local book store in the early 1970s McGrady, a columnist on the Long Island paper *Newsday*, observed that the bestsellers were the books that contained sex – lots of it. McGrady thought it was pretty depressing and wanted to do something about it. The other journalists he spoke to agreed that it was trash that people seemed to want. It wasn't long before they'd cooked up a scheme to write a novel of such uniform dreadfulness that the others would be shown up for what they were.

McGrady organized the project and laid down a few simple instructions for the others to follow. There were twenty-four writers in total, each contributing a chapter with a minimum of two sexual encounters – the more and the kinkier the better. Anything remotely like good writing was ruthlessly cut, and in three weeks this catalogue of sex in suburbia, titled *Naked Came the Stranger*, was ready. It bore the name Penelope Ashe.

Within hours of receiving the manuscript the publishers were on the telephone. The book was amazing. Could Ms Ashe appear on TV to help promote it? Could she just! McGrady lined up his sister-in-law, an attractive lady in her twenties, to play the part of Penelope Ashe. Dressed in the tight trousers and plunging blouse that one might expect of suburban sex maniacs, she carried it off perfectly, right to the edge of parody. But instead of being rumbled as a spoof, *Naked Came the Stranger* began to gather a terrible momentum. Three days after publication it had sold twenty thousand copies and negotiations were under way for the film rights. McGrady and his fellow writers were finally forced to admit that there was nothing so dreadful that the American public wouldn't go crazy for it.

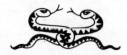

In the annals of sex education Armpitin doesn't get much of a mention, but it had a brief moment of glory when it was the subject of a paper written by a Canadian physician, J. S. Greenstein. At the heart of the excitement lay its chemical formula, which Dr Greenstein explained contained several groups of molecules identified by the initials NO. Tests revealed that the new contraceptive worked on the male sense of smell and via the olfactory nerves made the user impotent for a number of days equivalent to the number of NO molecular groups in the formula.

The paper received quite a few reviews in medical journals and several drug companies knocked on Dr Greenstein's door to buy the patent from him. He was left to explain that Armpitin was a hoax.

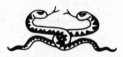

When Allan and Sheila MacGregor waved goodbye to their families and set off for the Lake District for their honeymoon, both were looking forward to the privacy of two weeks together. Allan had five younger brothers and Sheila was from a large family too, so they hadn't had much chance to be alone during their engagement. By the time they drove up outside their honeymoon hotel the young lovers could scarcely keep their hands off each other, but they did their best to look nonchalant as they checked in at reception. They'd made it up to their room without being rumbled as newly-weds and were just beginning to do what honeymooners are supposed to do when there was a knock at the door. Champagne? Flowers? A surprise present? Not exactly. It was Sheila's parents, who were so worried about their daughter, who'd never spent a night away from them before, that they'd decided to come on the honeymoon too.

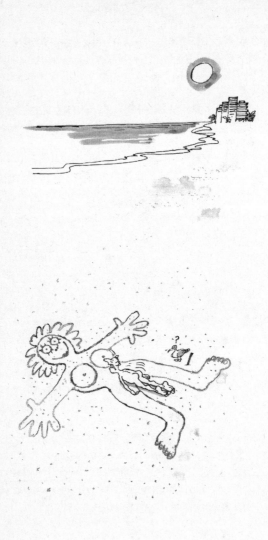

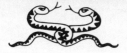

Ellen Gross from Chicago was enjoying a drink in a bar with a girlfriend when she looked across the room and spotted the man who was made for her. 'It was instant attraction,' she revealed in a newspaper interview. 'He looked great and I thought, that's the one for me. He seemed to feel the same way too, because he came over and we began talking, and we had the same interests and everything. It was perfect. When he heard it was my birthday coming up the next week he said, "Why don't we celebrate by getting married?" So we did.' What came next was a terrible surprise, because on their first night together her ideal man turned out to be not so perfect; he was a woman. Mrs Gross took it on the chin and decided to try to make it work. 'Naturally I feel I've been cheated, but the relationship has given a whole new dimension to my life. Before I married Ron I wouldn't have dreamed of sleeping with a woman. Now I'm getting much more adaptable.'

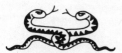

One is fun, they say, but thirty-three-year-old Mike Eastwood had an unpleasant surprise when he went on a holiday that had as its slogan, 'Sand, sea and fun in the sun on our sexy singles weeks.' It really *was* a singles holiday. Mike was the only one who booked it and he spent a fortnight on Ibiza making his own fun.

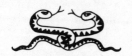

In these liberated days it's fine to go out looking for sex, and plenty of it. But fifty years ago a happily married man could be forgiven for worrying if he was getting too much of a good thing. A Mr Dittrick, described as 'mentally bright, capable and a good worker', found himself up in court in Minnesota accused of being a sexual psychopath. His crime? He was reckoned to have an unnatural sexual appetite for his wife's favours. The prosecution estimated that Mr Dittrick liked to have sex three or four times a week and this was considered so excessive that he was duly put away.

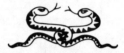

Another man who liked sex was Gaetan le Guillou, a French forestry worker who felt under the weather and went to his doctor complaining of dizzy spells. The doctor's tests revealed that he was suffering from a drug overdose, which came as a surprise to Gaetan as he wasn't taking drugs. Then Madame le Guillou owned up. She had been slipping tranquillizers into his food to try to curb his sexual appetite.

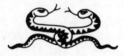

New Yorker Robert Stuart decided to give his girlfriend a surprise when she jilted him. He called at her house, stood on the doorstep, stuck a 'super-blockbuster' firework in his mouth and lit it. The resulting explosion certainly made his point. His girlfriend was taken to hospital in a state of shock. There wasn't enough of Robert left to make a trip to the hospital worth while for him.

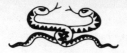

Another excitable New Yorker, Zaza Kimmont, got back from a trip only to discover a strange toothbrush lying beside her husband's in the bathroom. On close inspection it proved to have a trace of lipstick on the bristles. Zaza's jealous rage was uncontrollable. She swept through the house smashing everything she could get her hands on, upending furniture and causing more than £5000-worth of damage. Then she packed a bag and went to her mother's, where a surprise was waiting for her. Her mother knew all about the other woman; she was Zaza's mother-in-law, who had been to stay at the flat while she was away and had left her toothbrush behind . . .

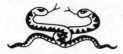

Of all Europeans the Italians are supposed to be the most hot-blooded and Evaristo Bertone, an eighty-five-year-old Sicilian, certainly lived up to the national reputation when he found a love letter that had been sent to his wife Adriana. Mad with jealousy and the idea that she had been unfaithful, he stabbed her in the shoulder. This was all something of a surprise to Adriana, who asked to see the letter. When he showed it to her she tactfully pointed out that he had written it himself, fifty years ago. 'His eyesight is so poor that I forgave him,' she said.

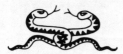

Also in trouble over love letters was Trudy Hochman from Illinois. When her boyfriend Wayne came across three steamy love notes in the glove compartment of her car he went wild and smashed the windscreen and let down the tyres. Then he went looking for Trudy and gave her a black eye. Before he could do anything more the police intervened and arrested him. They wanted to take a look at the love letters as evidence against him but Trudy was reluctant to hand them over. The reason became clear when Wayne made his court appearance. Trudy, fearing that he didn't love her, had written them herself and hidden them in the car. 'I guess I can only blame myself,' she said, emerging from the court with Wayne, who'd been fined. 'It was a small price to pay to know how much Wayne really loves me.'

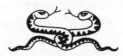

While we're on the subject of love and hoaxes, let's take a look at Valentine's Day. Perhaps it's time to reveal that for around five hundred years we've been conned about that most romantic of saints. According to Professor Henry Kelly, who has spent eight years studying the origins of the tradition, we're celebrating the wrong saint on the wrong day. The Valentine we *should* be remembering is St Valentine of Genoa, who died on 3 May. And when you think about it there's more sense in having a day devoted to lovers in spring, when a young man's fancy really does turn to thoughts of love, than in February when all his fancy can rise to is a bowl of soup and a hot water bottle.

So who's to blame for this particular sexual disaster? Professor Kelly lays the blame on Queen Isobel of Bavaria, who launched a Charter of the Court of Love – a sort of medieval escort agency – and set it on 'the day of my Lord St Valentine'. She chose the wrong saint and therefore the wrong day, and we've been celebrating the error ever since.

The party's
over

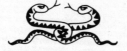

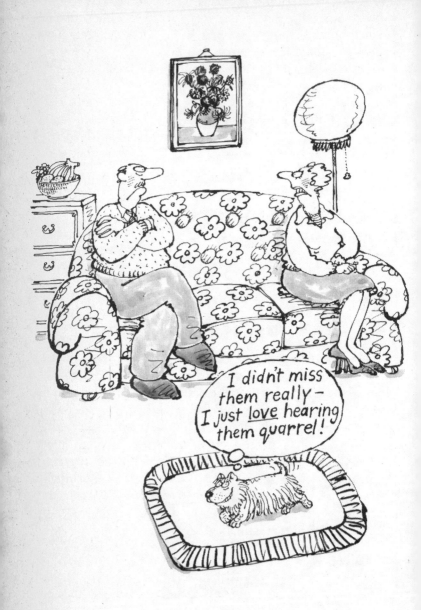

Determined to do things properly were Carey and Yvonne McCormack who filed for divorce in 1984. They made civilized agreements about their home and contents and financial support for Yvonne, but when it came to Pilchard, their West Highland terrier, they simply couldn't come to an arrangement. He had been a gift from Carey on their first wedding anniversary and they both loved him very much. After an attempt at sharing him, one week with Carey and the next with Yvonne, Pilchard started to pine and they were forced to admit that the emotional upheaval was too much for him. In despair, neither willing to give him up, they moved in together and after a few weeks were back as man and wife. 'This doesn't mean that we won't eventually divorce,' insisted a sheepish Carey, 'but while Pilchard's alive we won't be splitting up.' A vet estimated that they could look forward to at least another ten years of married life.

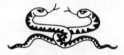

Joseph Kagari found that the best way of enticing Filipino girls into bed was to promise to marry them. His tactic seldom failed and each time he enjoyed himself for a few weeks before disappearing and leaving his 'fiancée' to pick up the pieces. Then he fell in love and decided to do it for real. His fiancée's parents were so pleased about the wedding that they put an announcement in the newspaper. On the great day Joseph arrived in church to be confronted by seven girls he'd already promised to marry, all of them armed with writs for breach of promise. He ran, and is reported to be running still.

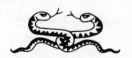

The Little White Chapel in Las Vegas, where *Dynasty* star Joan Collins plighted her troth for the fourth time in 1986, has removed and smashed the wall plaque commemorating this historic event. The owners said that the highly disputed divorce case that marked the end of the marriage would be bad for business.

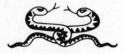

The cost of keeping his divorced wife Christina proved too much for New York psychiatrist Dr Edmondo Torres. He shot himself rather than face her constant demands for alimony, but not before he'd cut her out of his will. Christina heard of his death and the will in rapid succession and applied for the right to have her husband's ashes – so that she could flush them down the loo. Her petition was refused.

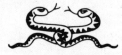

Another divorced husband devised a cunning way of getting his own back on his wife. Sefton Marks, a furrier from Solihull, was being pressured by his ex-wife who was anxious to receive the last instalment of her settlement. They finally agreed on a date and time that the payment was to be made. The day came and the hour passed. The ex-Mrs Sefton called her husband and his assistant assured her that the cash was on its way. And sure enough, it was. Only twenty minutes later an armoured van drew up and out stepped three helmeted guards each carrying a small sack. Mrs Marks was confused. How could £25,000 be fitted into just three small sacks? It couldn't, explained the guards – there were fifty more waiting in the van. Sefton had arranged to pay her in £1 coins and other assorted change.

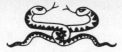

Feeling deflated after being let down by his girlfriend, who'd run off with a driving instructor, Alfonso Monta reaped his revenge through the streets of the Paraguayan capital Asunción by letting down the tyres of every parked car he came across. When police finally caught up with him he'd left hundreds of furious motorists stranded by the roadside.

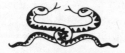

Hell hath no fury like a woman scorned, they say, but the revenge of a jealous husband can be pretty spectacular. Anna May Reese's estranged husband dedicated himself to violent revenge when she left him for a new man, and he vowed to do away with his rival. Between the springs of Anna May's bed he hid a stick of dynamite, running the fuse through a loose floorboard and out through the wall of the house. Thus prepared, he waited until the lovers were bonking beneath the sheets before lighting the fuse.

Unfortunately his research hadn't gone as far as checking their favoured positions for making love. Instead of being on top, Anna May was flat on her back in the bed when the explosion went off. She was killed while her boyfriend, who'd certainly felt the earth move, walked away scorched but otherwise uninjured.

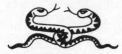

Peter the Great of Russia had an even more gruesome way of imposing fidelity on the women in his life. When one of his mistresses was unfaithful to him he had her head chopped off and pickled in alcohol. Then he kept it by the side of his bed as a reminder to the others of the fate that lay in wait for them if they strayed. To his wife he was a little more understanding. He didn't behead her but he *did* behead her lover, William Mons, and present her with his pickled head to keep beside her bed as a warning.

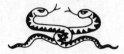

To celebrate the end of his first marriage an Esher man ordered a dozen cases of champagne from his wine merchant. Unfortunately he forgot to check whether the wine merchant had his latest address . . . and the bubbly was delivered to his old address where his ex-wife was able to celebrate at his expense.

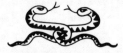

Following a row with his girlfriend, Francisco Cruz followed her in his car, pursuing her as she walked along the pavement. In an attempt to get away from him she rushed into a waterbed showroom – and he followed her, still in his car. Customers and staff dived for cover as the saloon smashed through the plate glass windows and slithered to a halt, bursting mattresses and flooding the ground floor. The Huntingdon Beach Police were called and booked Cruz for attempted murder, alleging that he had tried to murder the girl.

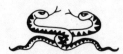

In the autumn of 1982 Adrian Barnes planted a romantic spring surprise for his girlfriend Pat, but their romance didn't last and they broke up before Christmas. Adrian

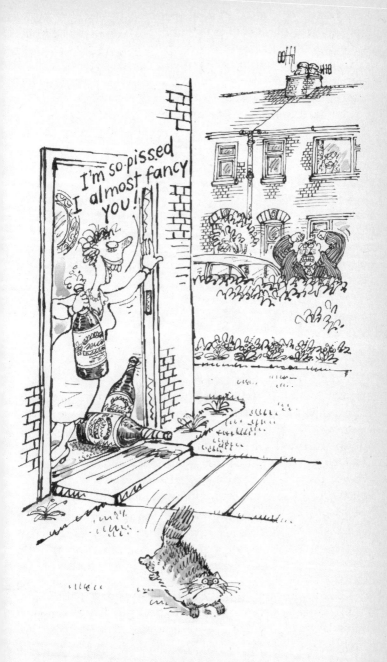

moved away and Pat thought she'd forgotten him. Then came spring – and with it two hundred yellow and white crocuses which sprouted on the front lawn of her home and spelled out the message, 'Pat, I love you for ever, Adrian', for everyone to see.

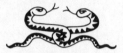

It was all over for George Baxter after a row with his wife in June 1965. He stormed out of the house to take the babysitter home vowing, 'When I get back I'll show you something.' And he did. On his return to the house he went out to the patio at the back and called his wife to come out. Brandishing a can of petrol he threatened to pour it over himself. 'Don't be silly,' she warned, stunned, but before she could do anything he'd doused himself and lit a match.

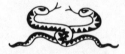

Despite the examples of bad behaviour, unhappiness and suffering that come before them every day in their work, some divorce court judges still seem to have a somewhat quaint and even old-fashioned view of marriage and morals. Giving a ruling on one divorce case, Judge Blagdon observed that a man who had received hospitality in his cousin's home and then misbehaved with the cousin's wife had done something which, in his opinion, was as morally reprehensible as stealing the silver spoons from the dining room. And in the USA Commissioner Bush James had obviously failed to keep abreast of the popularity of wife-swapping. 'For a husband to permit his wife to go committing adultery and then to go into the next room and himself commit adultery with his hostess seems to me an extraordinary piece of bad behaviour.'

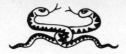

The party came to an abrupt end for the Reverend Harold Davidson, Vicar of Stiffkey, a tiny north Norfolk village, in the spring of 1932. He was hauled before a church court to answer charges relating to his private life – charges that held the whole country enthralled.

The good vicar had the habit of picking up young girls and offering them work in the film industry, according to the evidence of one of the young witnesses who had been approached by Davidson at Marble Arch and asked if she was a film actress. As she was only sixteen at the time this would have been unlikely. However, it served its purpose and they got talking. Before long she had been set up in a flat of her own and received regular night-time visits as part of the vicar's 'rescue work'.

While the court case was unfolding there were a number of strange events at Stiffkey, where new priests had been appointed to take over during the Reverend Davidson's absence. On one occasion the vicar returned and tried to take the morning and evening services himself. The locals were treated to the sight of the two clergymen tussling in the pulpit, each trying to grab the Bible. It was noted that the lady parishioners cheered on the Reverend Davidson, who was popular in the area.

When the guilty verdict came through no one was very surprised. Davidson had expected to be unfrocked and set about raising funds for an appeal. Among his stunts was an appearance sitting in a barrel on the promenade at Blackpool; he was arrested and fined for this display. The eccentric behaviour continued. Davidson even went to his own unfrocking at Norwich Cathedral and heckled the bishop. Back in Blackpool he exhibited himself in a glass case in which he was prodded by a mechanical devil. A sign on the outside of the case read, 'I am determined to fast until death.' The zealous policemen promptly arrested him for attempted suicide.

Two years later, and still in the quest for justice, he could be found in a lion's cage. Spectators willing to part with threepence witnessed the vicar standing next to a lion as he delivered a speech proclaiming his innocence. One day they got more of a spectacle than they'd bargained for, for the vicar stepped back on to the lion, which took exception to being trodden on and mauled him badly. As he was dragged clear and it became obvious that he would not survive, he asked what time it was. Three-thirty, someone told him. 'Ah, time to make the evening papers,' he commented before he died.

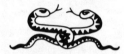

Back on the subject of divorce, few can rival the feat of Mr Alhaji Mohamed of Walworth, who was divorced by two wives in a period of fifteen minutes on 17 July 1975 at the High Court in London. As a Muslim, Mr Mohamed is entitled to up to four wives. The first divorce went to Mrs Adiza Mohamed, who had lived apart from her husband for two years, and just a few minutes later Mrs Rabi Mohamed obtained her decree, enabling her to marry someone else.

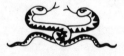

Divorce court regulars Dorothy and David Funk were back for their fifth divorce in 1970. Their fifth marriage had foundered after seven months and on this occasion it was Mrs Funk who filed for the decree. Their first marriage in 1950 had lasted for seven years before it was deemed to have broken down irreparably. Their subsequent divorces, all allowed on the same grounds, had been granted in 1962, 1964 and 1965.

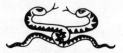

'My wife got the house, the car, the bank account, and if I marry again and have children, she gets them too,' observed Woody Allen. It's a sad fact that when the party's over it's those who've lived and loved to the full who have to pay most for their pleasure . . .

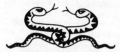

Take the example of John Stratton, who decided to kill himself when his wife left him. He sealed all the doors and windows of his house and turned on the gas oven. Unaware that it was non-toxic North Sea gas, he waited for it to take effect. It didn't, and while he was waiting he had time to reflect that maybe life wasn't so terrible after all. Perhaps he *could* struggle through. He celebrated this change of heart with a cigarette. He and half the house were blown to pieces.

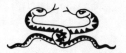

When Alice Nunn received notification that her husband Amin was suing her for divorce she was shocked. As far as she knew, she'd never been married and she certainly didn't know anyone called Amin. Investigations revealed that someone had obtained vital details about her from her birth certificate, which they'd applied for at Somerset House, and then used the information as a cover for their marriage. Alice's lawyer commiserated but could only suggest that she went through with the divorce. Six months later she was a single woman again – as she'd always been.

On the subject of extraordinary marriages, Giuseppe Garibaldi, the Italian leader, had one of the shortest on record. At the age of fifty-two he married his eighteen-year-old bride – only to discover, a few minutes after the ceremony, that she was not the innocent he had imagined. Her cousin, one Major Rovell, not only revealed that the lovely Giuseppina had been sleeping around since the age of eleven but that he had had the pleasure of her too. At this Garibaldi called his wife a whore and never spoke to her again. However, it was only twenty years later that they were formally divorced.

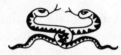

Wealthy businessman David Hirschmann was quite straight with his wife before they married. He wanted sex every night or he would sulk. Mrs Cherrie Hirschmann obviously thought he was joking because she went through with the wedding – but he wasn't. And after thirteen years of making love nightly or suffering, she went to the divorce court. If she'd only had to put up with sulking Mrs Hirschmann might not have minded, but when she said 'no' he expressed his disapproval by kicking her out of bed and beating her with a toy sword. Despite all this, Mr Hirschmann denied that he'd been insensitive to his wife's feelings; the judge disagreed.

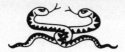

Eighty-four-year-old Michael Vira's problem was also one of sex. He filed a divorce suit in Manhattan Supreme Court alleging that Mrs Anna Vira had withdrawn conjugal rights from him for fifty-four years. His claim was correct, but there was rather more to it than met the eye as the court discovered when they considered Mrs Vira's counter-claim. She'd filed it from her home in Czechoslovakia – where she'd been living ever since Michael waved goodbye and went to the USA to make his fortune in 1926.

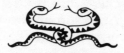

A divorce was granted on the grounds of cruelty to a Torbay lady in 1981. The court had heard that her husband was an insanely jealous man who had destroyed his wife's clothing and locked her in the house in his attempts to stop other men catching a glimpse of her. After this evidence, there was some consternation in court when she didn't turn up to hear the verdict. A police officer was sent with her husband, who swore he didn't know where she was, to look for her. She was found locked in the bathroom at their home.

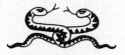

A divorce case that ended in failure involved Italian Attilio Gianti, who penned passionate and incriminating love letters to the married woman with whom he was having an affair. When the lady's husband sued for divorce, Attilio vowed to swallow his words – literally. He went

along to the office of her husband's lawyer and asked if he
could have one last look at the letters. As they were
handed to him he shoved them into his mouth and began
to chew. Before anyone could stop him he'd swallowed
the lot. Because, apart from a severe attack of indigestion,
there was no evidence, the judge dismissed the divorce
case.

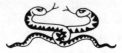

A romantic American couple called Valentine arranged to
receive their decree absolute on 14 February because, as
they said, 'It rounds the whole marriage off nicely.' Others
have found equally unusual ways of celebrating D-day
with as much style as they did their wedding day. Gene
and Lynda Ballard were divorced while freefalling at 120
miles per hour. A brave lawyer, who jumped out of the
aeroplane with them, served the divorce papers on Gene
at 12,000 feet. Then the high-flying couple dropped out of
each other's lives. Flying at roughly the same height when
she was divorced was a nameless Egyptian woman who
had a row with her husband at Cairo airport in 1986. The
husband, who remained on the ground, decided that he'd
had enough and solicited the help of the airport's control
tower to tell her 'I divorce thee' three times.

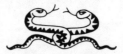

Rose and Antony Johnson decided to hold a 'Not a
Wedding' party to celebrate the end of their marriage in
November 1986. They invited everyone who'd been to
the original wedding and had such a good time that by the
end of the evening they'd decided to give it another go.

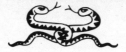

A trip to a travel agent's ended in divorce for a Nottingham woman. Her husband was flicking through the brochures she'd brought home when he spotted a picture of her lying topless in the Mediterranean sun with their next-door neighbour at her side. The wife owned up. More than a year before she'd squeezed in a trip to Spain while he'd been away on a training course. While her husband sued her for divorce, she tried to sue the travel company for using a photo they'd taken without permission.

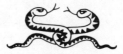

With lawyers trying to get the best they can for each of their clients, divorces between even the most civilized people can end up being acrimonious. Take the case of Eugene Schneider. When a judge ordered him to divide his property equally with his wife, Eugene took him at his word and sliced their wooden bungalow neatly down the middle with a chainsaw.

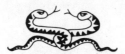

But it's not always divorce that puts an end to the good times. Richard 'Beau' Nash, the self-styled King of Bath who was famed for his eccentric behaviour, died in 1761 and left a distraught mistress. She vowed that she would never sleep in a bed again, and she was true to her word. Near Bishopstrow, Wiltshire, she found a huge hollowed-out tree in which she made her home. She lived there for the next seventeen years.